THE NEW
BODY
BOOK

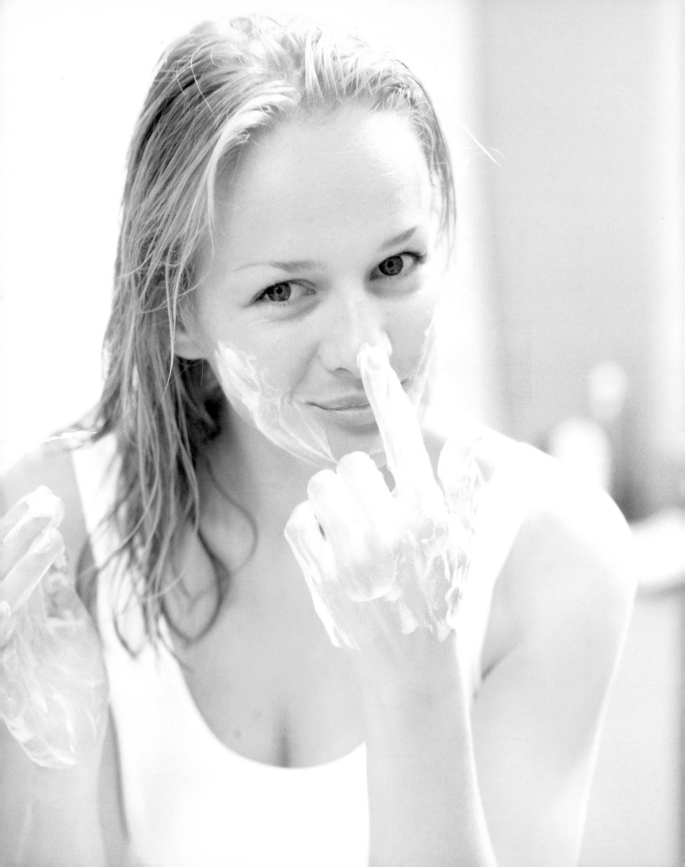

THE NEW
BODY
BOOK

Nicola Moulton

APPLE

Apple Press

Sheridan House

112–116A Western Road

Hove

East Sussex BN3 1DD

UK

Text and design copyright © The Ivy Press Limited 2003

This book was conceived, designed and produced by

The Ivy Press Limited, The Old Candlemakers, Lewes, East Sussex BN7 2NZ, U.K.

Creative director Peter Bridgewater

Publisher Sophie Collins

Editorial director Steve Luck

Design manager Tony Seddon

Art director Clare Barber

Senior project editor Caroline Earle

Illustrations Emma Brownjohn

Picture research Liz Eddison

Every effort has been taken to ensure that all information in this book is correct. This book is not intended to replace consultation with your doctor, surgeon or other healthcare professional. The author and publisher disclaim any liability, loss, injury or damage incurred as a consequence, directly or indirectly, of the use and application of the contents of this book.

ISBN: 1 84092 392 X

A CIP catalogue record for this book is available from the British Library

Printed in China by Hong Kong Graphics and Printing Ltd.

Contents

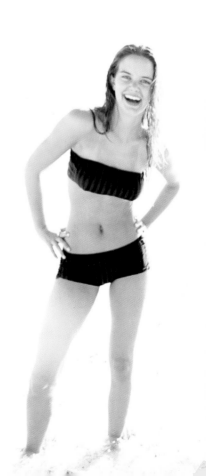

introduction

There's nothing stopping you from having the best body you possibly can – all it takes is a little knowledge, a lot of effort and a very large helping of attitude. Offering a balanced view of diet and lifestyle, exercise, treatments and cosmetic surgery, *The New Body Book* will set you off on the right track to a fit, firm and healthy body. Here's how.

THIS WAY TO A BETTER BODY

Unless you happen to be a supermodel with enviable pro-portions (and let's face it, there are only about five of those in the world), we all need to lavish a little attention on our bodies from time to time. *The New Body Book* is for those very times. It's designed to give you hope, motivation and inspiration whether you're planning on doing a short burst of intensive training to get into shape for a special occasion, or want a meticulously planned beauty regime that will overhaul your whole body.

Guiding you through each part of the body, working from the top right down to your toes, each section looks at a different body part and contains everything you need to know about your diet, exercise regime, beauty products and treatments, and surgery options. The guiding principle behind the book is that while it's not normally possible to 'spot treat' different areas of the body, it's certainly true that each body part responds differently to various treatments and routines. These days, research into health and beauty has become so specific that it's possible to tailor the foods you eat, the exercise you take and the beauty products you choose to what it is about your body that you most want to change. The trick is to know exactly what's right for you – and that's where *The New Body Book* comes in.

Once you have worked out where your dream body and real physique can meet, then you can start optimising your potential. When it comes to improving your arms, for example, weights and repetition exercises will give you a strong, muscular appearance, while stretching regimes such as yoga can give arms a lean, streamlined look. If it's your legs that you're targeting, it's useful to know that you can now get creams and lotions that have been created specifically for soothing and re-energising tired legs, containing synthetic ingredients that feel cool on the skin and natural soothers such as menthol and aloe. If it's your complexion you're worried about, perhaps you need help cutting through the masses of information about the various injec-tions and non-surgical procedures available.

On top of a comprehensive low-down on how each body part works, there's also an important emphasis on the new. Each section will leave you fully versed in the latest products, the newest procedures and the most current thinking. As with most things, sometimes the latest developments prove to be invaluable, other times it's the tried-and-tested approach that turns out to be best. Either way, the most important thing is to familiarize yourself with what's out there – so you can choose the option that appeals to you most.

All the information is presented in a clear, easy-to-understand format with advice and tips from experts in each field. Reading the book should be a bit like having a personal shopper for your body – someone who knows all the latest research, and can edit down the bits you need so that you don't have to spend time wading through mountains of irrelevant information. Simply turn to the section that you're interested in, find exactly the right body part, choose which of the areas (diet, exercise, beauty treatments or surgery) you want to look at first and you're away. And because of the synergistic nature of your body, you'll find that each section leads naturally onto others so that before you know it you'll have read up on an entire section.

However, all that knowledge isn't going to go very far if you're still not tempted to put it to good use. That's why there's an entire section devoted to wellbeing – a very important area when it comes to looking after your body. In this section you'll find advice on how to get started, things to do when you've been following the same routine for a while and feel that you've 'plateaued', and also ways to improve your confidence and feel better about yourself while you're still on the road to a better body.

Improving your fitness and enhancing your appearance shouldn't be the hard slog that we all fear it's going to be – with the right attitude, it can be a walk in the park, so read on and make the decision to begin your walk in the park today.

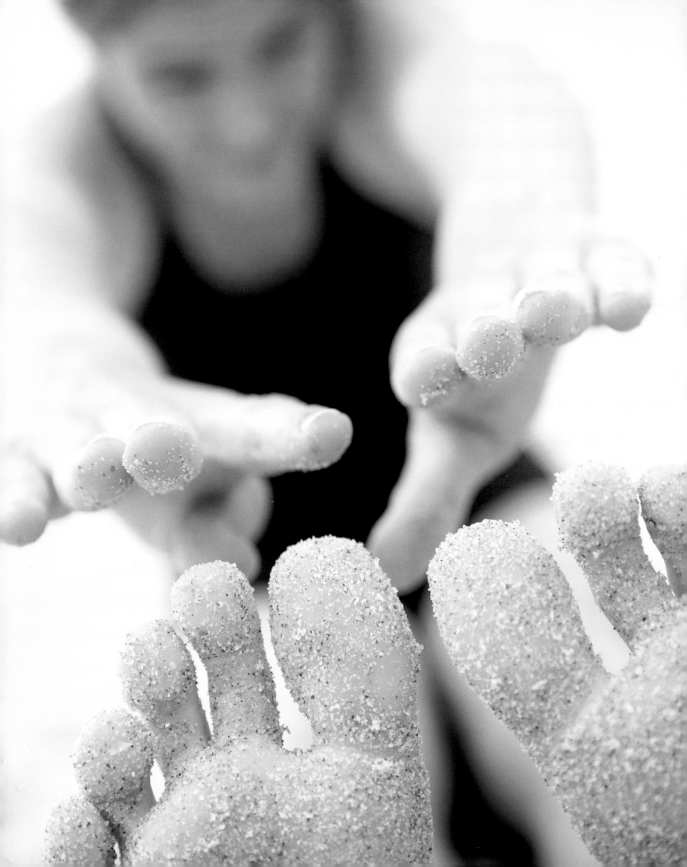

body

Achieving a smoother, firmer, younger-looking body must be the holy grail for every woman. Even if you're not a beauty addict or eager to try out the latest fitness fads, there are still untold benefits to be reaped from knowing which foods will give you long-term energy and which stretching exercises will improve your posture and keep your joints more supple. Recently, the health and beauty industries have harnessed the trend for all things 'holistic', a word literally meaning 'whole'. The theory goes that in order to get the best from our bodies, we have to treat each part of ourselves as an individual piece in a bigger puzzle. This opening section will do just that. It takes the 'puzzle' out of getting a better body and shows you how to adopt, piece by piece, a modern approach to diet, fitness, beauty and cosmetic surgery, changing the body you have into the body you want.

fit to be eaten

When talking about a better body, it's impossible not to start with food, and with the fabulous array of ever-more exotic tastes and textures now available to us, meals have never been more varied – or more tempting. So before you allow your appetite to run riot, read on and give some thought to which nutrients your body really needs on a daily basis.

NEW WAYS TO EAT YOURSELF HEALTHY

We are all aware that the ideal scenario is to eat what you need in order to stay healthy, and secondly to enjoy what you eat, but the trick is to make the two things match up. This is partly a question of appetite. The way that most of us eat whenever food is offered – whether hungry or not – stems back, scientists say, to our ancestors, who came across food so sporadically that they ate their fill whenever it was available. This means that in today's plentiful world, we have to retrain ourselves to eat only when hungry. A good tip is to ask yourself what you feel like eating. Research shows that if you're truly hungry, you'll be equally as happy eating an apple as you will a chocolate bar, but if you're eating out of boredom, the apple won't seem so appealing.

CONTROL YOUR WEIGHT

It's also important to distinguish dieting from eating healthily. In a nutshell, dieting is for weight loss, and healthy eating is for long-term energy (though a sensible weight-loss diet won't leave you lethargic). Both should cover the right quantities of all the food groups – see the diagram opposite. Most women want to keep weight down – it's thought that one in four Western women are on a weight-loss programme at any given time – but some want to maintain, or even increase, their weight (in order to conceive, for example). Studies have shown that meal replacement systems (which use specially formulated thick shakes or snack bars) actually work better than food alone as a weight maintenance strategy. Simply replace one meal a day instead of the two suggested for weight loss. Plus, a touch of extra weight might not be the health hazard we once thought. Surveys have shown that slightly overweight women (up to around 8 lbs/3.6 kilos) tend to live longer than their thinner counterparts.

Losing weight becomes more of an issue as we get older, with the average woman gaining around $1\frac{1}{2}$ lbs (675 grams) every year after the age of thirty-five. What's more, in advancing years, that weight becomes harder to shift. This means that successful weight-loss programmes should not just be about eating less, but should also incorporate a change in exercise and lifestyle patterns. Reducing caloric intake alone will take longer, won't last and will not result in a well-toned body. Exercise not only burns calories; it also builds muscles, puts you in a better mood and improves your cardiovascular and bone health. At the very least, it should be the partner of calorie reduction, but in truth it is more important and more effective in lasting weight loss than counting calories ever could be.

MIRACLE SOLUTIONS?

Not surprisingly, many women are turning to more extreme methods of weight loss. Fad diets are common, but potentially dangerous. For example, both the 'all-fruit' and the 'no carbs' diets produce dramatic weight loss at first, but what you're losing is mostly water, so it's weight you'll quickly gain back. At the same time, any diet that excludes one of the major food groups (and carbohydrates are the most important one for total body health) is depriving you of health-promoting antioxidants and phytochemicals, fibre, vitamins and minerals.

Appetite-suppressant tablets are also on the increase, but these tablets should be approached with caution. The 'stimulant' variety can be addictive and may be dangerous for people who have high blood pressure, heart conditions, diabetes, thyroid disease or kidney problems. The 'laxative' type can cause damage to the colon and also prevent you from getting the full benefit from many of the nutrients in your food, and in any case will not help lose body fat. Other, more extreme methods include jaw-wiring, which restricts food intake; stomach stapling, which reduces stomach size, meaning that it's impossible to overeat; and intestinal bypass, which prevents the absorption of food. These are normally turned to only in cases of severe obesity and should always be arranged by a certified physician.

What you need to get by

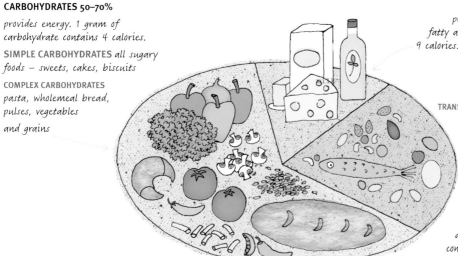

CARBOHYDRATES 50–70%

provides energy. 1 gram of carbohydrate contains 4 calories.

SIMPLE CARBOHYDRATES *all sugary foods – sweets, cakes, biscuits*

COMPLEX CARBOHYDRATES *pasta, wholemeal bread, pulses, vegetables and grains*

FACT 10% of our daily energy is taken up processing our food.

FAT 20–30%
provides energy and essential fatty acids. 1 gram of fat contains 9 calories. Keep saturated and trans-fats to a minimum.

SATURATED *butter, cheese, full cream milk*

TRANS-FATS *labelled 'hydrogenated fat' on margarine, baked goods and snack foods*

UNSATURATED *vegetable oils, nuts, seeds, oily fish*

PROTEIN 20–30%
provides amino acids – the building blocks for growth and repair. 1 gram of protein contains 4 calories. Eat it every day – your body can't store it.

HIGH BIOLOGICAL *adequate amounts of essential amino acids – meat, fish, eggs*

LOW BIOLOGICAL *inadequate amounts of essential amino acids – pulses, nuts, seeds*

THE LOWDOWN ON ESSENTIAL EXTRAS

We are supposed to drink at least 2 litres ($4\tfrac{1}{4}$ pints) of water every day, but most people don't understand why. Among other things, water is essential for keeping our digestive system ticking over properly, eliminating toxins, lubricating our joints and eyes, keeping skin supple and helping to protect our nervous system. And it's essential for keeping our bodies in shape – it suppresses the appetite and helps the liver and kidneys to function properly.

WATER FACTS

The sensation of thirst is not triggered until there is already a water deficit, so drink before you get thirsty. The 2-litre requirement is for plain water, not coffee, tea, soft drinks, soup and other watery foods. Some contain salt, which increases the water requirement, and/or have diuretic properties (coffee and tea, for example), which promote fluid loss. Not all waters are the same. Levels of minerals

WATER BABE *Believe it or not, water makes up about one half of your entire body, and fully 75 per cent of your brain!*

vary between sources, so rely on your diet as a source of minerals and trace elements, not water. Water retention isn't a problem of excess water – it's more likely to be a problem of excess salt. Keep drinking your 2 litres!

SUPPLEMENTARY BENEFITS?

How necessary are vitamin and mineral supplements? Medical and nutritional experts contend that the best source of needed micronutrients (vitamins and minerals) is a balanced diet. If you are concerned that you're not getting enough from your daily diet, you can safely take a single multivitamin-mineral tablet a day, which will contain all the important ones in the proper proportions. It is not recommended to take individual micronutrient tablets, and certainly not 'megadoses' of them.

There are exceptions. The elderly and people who smoke and drink a great deal of alcohol often do not get the nutrients they need from food, and could benefit from a single daily vitamin-mineral supplement. Strict vegetarians and vegans do not get enough vitamin B12 (found in animal protein) so they should take a B12 supplement. To prevent serious birth defects, women of childbearing age should take a folic acid supplement before attempting to become pregnant, and a multivitamin-mineral supplement formulated for pregnancy as soon as they get the news. Women who have experienced the menopause should take extra calcium (up to 1,500mg a day) to prevent the loss of bone density that leads to osteoporosis. In order to process calcium properly, the body needs vitamin D. That's why many calcium supplements also come with vitamin D, added in just the right proportion.

A new area of research, chemoprevention, is investigating whether vitamins and minerals can help prevent illnesses ranging from cancer to dementia. Studies are being done, but nothing conclusive has been found yet. If you want to add to the micronutrients in your diet with supplemental pills, be sure you don't exceed the RDA (*see chart*), especially of the fat-soluble vitamins (such as vitamins A, D, E and K), which are stored in the body and can build up to toxic levels. Absorbing an excess of some nutrients may affect the absorption of certain others. For example, high doses of vitamin E can interfere with vitamin K absorption and high calcium can inhibit the action of iron, and zinc hinders the status of copper. High doses should therefore not be undertaken without consulting a doctor.

Multivitamins and minerals

THE prevailing medical opinion is that there is little scietific evidence of the benefits of multivitamins to the average person, but there is also little evidence of harm (where amounts do not exceed 100 per cent of the Recommended Dietary Allowances – RDA). Indeed, multivitamins could be particularly useful for someone on a weight-loss programme.

Key *mg = milligrams, mcg = micrograms*

Vitamin	RDA	Food source	Vitamin	RDA	Food source
Vitamin A	600mcg	Fortified milk, eggs, beef, chicken, carrots, apricots	Vitamin E	10mg	Sunflower seeds, whole grains, nuts, vegetable oils, avocados
Vitamin B6	1.2mg	Poultry, fish, soya, whole grains, nuts, seeds, bananas	Folic acid (B9)	400mcg	Leafy greens, pulses, fortified cereals/grain products
Vitamin B12	1.5mcg	Meat, fish, poultry, eggs, dairy	Phosphorous	550mg	Meat, fish, whole grains, cheese, nuts
Thiamine (B1)	0.8mg	Wheatgerm, soya beans, brown rice, nuts	Calcium	700mg	Milk, cheese, broccoli, fortified juices, sesame seeds
Riboflavin (B2)	1.1mg	Milk, eggs, fortified cereals, ice cream	Magnesium	300mg	Leafy greens, brown rice, nuts, whole grains
Niacin (B3)	13mg	Lean meat, fish, eggs, cheese, soya beans, nuts	Iron	14.8mg	Red meat, fish, poultry, fortified grain products
Pantothenic acid	6mg	Yeast, offal, brown rice, eggs, whole grains	Zinc	9.5mg	Shellfish, meat, poultry, pulses, nuts
Vitamin C	40mg	Citrus, leafy greens, tomatoes, peppers, potatoes	Iodine	140mcg	Seafood, pineapple, raisins, dairy produce, iodised salt
Vitamin D	5mcg	Dairy products, oily fish, eggs, sunlight	Selenium	75mcg	Wheatgerm, tuna, onions, tomatoes, broccoli

survival of the fittest

Taking exercise needn't be a chore we dread – and it won't give us muscles like a body-builder, either. We should always remember the benefits: regular exercise decreases our risk of heart disease and cancer, increases our strength, improves our body shape and gives us an added boost of self-confidence. So what's the problem?

AVOIDING EXERCISE

It's much easier to find half an hour in the day to call a friend or watch your favourite soap than it is to do thirty minutes' exercise. Current guidelines state that we should try to get at least that amount of physical activity on most

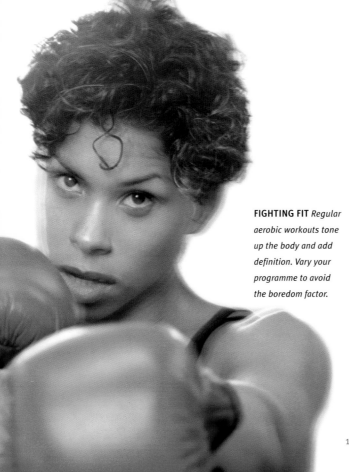

FIGHTING FIT *Regular aerobic workouts tone up the body and add definition. Vary your programme to avoid the boredom factor.*

– preferably all – days of the week, but with hectic schedules and families to take care of, there never seem to be enough hours in the day.

For many women, it's the thought of a frenzied workout in the gym that renders exercise so unappealing. The good news is that the days when fitness experts advocated 'pumping iron' and 'no pain, no gain' are long gone. Current thinking says that we can get all the exercise we need to keep our bodies healthy from only moderately strenuous activities such as a brisk walk or a gentle swim. Of course, if you want to be fit enough to run a marathon or go on a trekking holiday, you'll need to be doing more intensive cardiovascular workouts, but otherwise – it's no sweat.

One of the biggest myths surrounding exercise is that weight-training workouts give you masculine-looking weighty arms and bulky calves. They don't. Yes, they'll 'pump up' your muscles, but you'd need to be following the training and eating regimes of body-builders to achieve the same larger-than-life effect. What weight training does deliver is tone, because your muscles shorten as you use them, then elongate afterwards, so they're being exercised and sharpened. With stretching exercises such as yoga, you get the same effect but in reverse: muscles are elongated during the postures, then shorten when you've finished.

In both systems, the important point is that you've given your muscles a workout, strengthening and toning them, and improving your flexibility. The knock-on effect is a fitter, shapelier body: muscle burns far more calories than fat. Finally, when it comes to getting a shapelier body, no one way is best: ideally your fitness programme should be as varied as your lifestyle, meaning you'll need a combination of resistance (or weight) training, aerobic exercises and stretching. This fitness cocktail has another great advantage: with all those different things to do, there's little chance of you getting bored.

There are also recent studies to show that your personality can help dictate which kind of exercise is best for you. If you're methodical by nature, for example, you might get most satisfaction from exercises like swimming, where you can count the lengths. If you're naturally competitive, opt for team sports or classes where you're encouraged to measure your success against that of others. Alternatively, if you're a self-confessed sport-loather, try activities that get you fit by stealth – a Frisbee game in the park, for example, or 'dancercise' classes like jazz dance or salsa.

Another highly motivating factor comes courtesy of something all women love – shopping. Treating yourself to new fitness gear may make the difference between making an extra visit to the gym or ditching it for a night in front of the TV. Staple workout pieces such as trainers and sports bras shouldn't be changed too often – it's better to invest in one good item than several cheaper ones – but having an array of funky tops or brightly coloured shorts to show off could be just the enticement you need.

Types of exercise

Cardiovascular (aerobic) exercise

Cardiovascular exercise should occupy most of your fitness time.

Benefits Helps strengthen the heart and lungs and lower blood pressure and cholesterol. It increases stamina, meaning you don't get out of breath so easily.

Activities Walking, swimming, jogging, skipping, stair climbing, skiing, rowing, tae bo, cycling and spinning.

Frequency Five days out of seven for thirty minutes.

Strengthening exercise

Traditional notions of 'exercise routines' usually originate here – but it needn't be the never-ending agony you fear.

Benefits Builds muscle strength, boosting metabolism and giving tone and firmness to the body.

Activities Push-ups, stomach crunches, pull-ups, free weights and leg lifts.

Frequency Two twenty-minute workouts a week.

Stretching exercise

The most relaxing, is-this-really-work? discipline of the three – although you usually feel the effects the day after!

Benefits Increases the range of joints, making it easier to move about freely and without pain. It can also diminish your chance of causing joint and muscle injury.

Activities Yoga, Pilates, tai chi.

Frequency As often as you like. People find the more they stretch, the more they want to stretch.

AEROBIC EXERCISE

So you're embarking on a fitness regime? Eighty per cent of your routine should consist of cardiovascular exercise. Here's what you need to know...

IN THE BEGINNING

Aerobic means any sustained physical activity that increases the supply of oxygen, and therefore energy, to your muscles. That is, it's the kind of exercise that ups your heart rate and makes you breathe deeper and faster. Most fitness experts advise a minimum of twenty to thirty minutes of aerobic exercise per session. Aerobic exercises range from jogging, treadmills and elliptical trainers to step aerobic or dance classes. Strength training (using free weights and weight machines) is anaerobic exercise. Both burn calories, but aerobic exercise is more beneficial to the cardiovascular system.

If you're just starting out, it's advisable to work with a personal trainer who can get you started on a safe, individually tailored programme so you don't push yourself too hard and end up sore and discouraged. There's a broad range of activities that qualify as aerobic exercise. The important thing is to find out what you most like doing, and the only way to do that is to try.

STRENGTH OR STAMINA?

Once you've been exercising for six or eight sessions, it's normally about time to increase the intensity of your workout. You can do this in one of two ways: by increasing your strength, by walking up a steeper hill than usual, say, or setting the exercise bike a couple of notches harder; or by increasing your stamina, which simply involves carrying on exercising for longer than you were before. In these early stages, increasing your stamina is always advised: if the weights are too heavy, it's the skeletal system that takes the strain and you could end up injuring your knees, hips, shoulders, neck or back.

However, many fitness trainers now advocate 'interval training', where, as you exercise, you alternate between periods of high intensity and low intensity and build both your strength and stamina at once. For example, you could run for three minutes, walk for one minute, then run again, and so on, or you could swim five lengths at a brisk pace and then use a float to help with the next six. In the gym, treadmills and similar machines often have a 'random' setting that will automatically vary your workout intensity for you, and running in the countryside often provides a natural kind of interval training because of variations in the terrain.

These early stages of aerobic exercise, when you're just beginning to see results, are crucial. If you've been exercising for only a few weeks and then you miss, say, one week's worth of aerobic activity, it will take you several weeks to regain the standard you had reached. When your fitness has increased substantially, missing a couple of sessions won't have such a dramatic effect. Your psychological wellbeing is precarious at this stage, too: you won't be seeing real results yet and it's easy to get despondent. Increasing either the time or the distance of your workout by around 10 per cent a week will help this – you'll feel as if you're coming on in leaps and bounds and, before long, you will be.

Complete cardio guide

THE NEW AEROBICS Forget legwarmers, garish leotards and disco music. The new aerobics classes are fast, fun and varied – the idea is that you don't have time to feel tired...

Beginners

Water Workout Water provides such excellent resistance that the toning effects can be really effective – and you're exercising properly without getting all hot and sweaty.

Great for pregnant women and anyone who needs to protect her joints, because of arthritis, carpal tunnel syndrome, back or knee problems or other musculoskeletal conditions.

Tae Bo Think 'martial arts to music' and you've got the picture. This is a fantastic, fun class, where karate-style kicks and punches are combined with jazzy dance moves. Tae bo

is particularly good for improving general fitness – you don't spend much time working on individual body parts. A good, modern alternative to traditional aerobics.

Getting fitter

Spinning Forget wooden tops, we're talking about spinning bicycle wheels here. Each member of the class sits on a bicycle, and goes through a series of (stationary) sprints, races and hill

rides. Great for working the legs, and also a serious cardiovascular workout. Instructors always check participants' general level of fitness beforehand, because it's not for the new-to-exercise.

Boxercise™ Where tae bo borrows from martial arts, boxercise borrows from...boxing, although it's non-contact so you won't end up with a black eye! It combines boxing methods and

techniques with aerobics and fitness training, giving you an aerobic and anaerobic workout while improving flexibility and balance. Particularly good for the upper body.

Pretty fit

Body Pump This class is designed to be an intense gym-style workout combining aerobic and anaerobic exercise for those who don't like going to the gym. The exercises are quite static but

also very varied, using a mixture of free weight and body weight exercises, and each one is usually repeated substantially. Each major muscle group gets a good workout – it can be a pretty tough class.

Boot Camp As the name suggests, Boot Camp is military-style exercise such as sit-ups and squat thrusts, which you perform in a circuit. There was a craze for military-style

instructors barking orders at the class, and many of the originators were ex-army, but these days classes are less intimidating – though still physically quite demanding.

GET FLEXIBLE

Everyone can benefit from stretching. For those who exercise regularly, it's an excellent preliminary to any aerobic or weight-training session. It can also work wonders on its own. For those who are overweight or new to exercise, it's a safe and simple way to begin. Initially, stretches work best on muscles that are already fairly defined, so if you have a lot of weight to lose, it could take a good few months before you see tangible results.

It's a good idea to work with an instructor when beginning any stretching routine. If you over-stretch a muscle, you might tear or bruise it. Likewise, wrist, ankle or knee injuries can be made worse by too much or the wrong kind of stretching. Yoga is one very popular way to stretch.

It also emphasises breathing and balance. It can be done by beginners, who should start slowly with a few simple poses and gradually move on to more challenging ones.

So, after a stretching class, will you feel relaxed or invigorated? The good thing about stretching is that you get to decide. If you're at the end of a stressful day, a stretching session will help you relax. If you start your day with a stretch class, getting all that well-oxygenated blood to your muscles will give you the energy to cope with the day ahead.

TWO GOOD REASONS TO STRETCH

1. Stretching encourages good posture, which can benefit you in several ways. From the standpoint of health, it keeps your body in alignment, which minimises aches and pains,

Four great ways to stretch

Yoga Yoga literally means 'to yoke' – to join together mind, body and breath. When yoga came into being in northern India around 5,000 years ago, it was used to prepare the body for meditation. As well as being profoundly relaxing, it increases flexibility, strength, balance and co-ordination. There are many different schools of yoga, though all combine breathing, stretching and balance to achieve a series of postures, or asanas. Recently growing in popularity is 'power yoga', which is drawn from Ashtanga techniques and can be quite physically demanding. Even if you try yoga mainly for its relaxing and meditative benefits, you will get a good stretch in the process. You concentrate on each pose for a long time – it's not uncommon for a whole class to be based around one position. Regular practice will improve circulation and digestion and decrease the risk of joint complaints and asthma.

Pilates The new kid on the block so far as stretch classes are concerned, it was originally invented by Joseph Pilates to help injured dancers regain their physical strength. Breathing is central to Pilates and is different from most forms of exercise in that you breathe in, not out, when your body's doing the work. Expect to see an improvement in your posture, breathing, flexibility and, in particular, your abdominal muscles.

Aikido Aikido is a 20th-century Japanese system of harmony and wellbeing that was developed by Morihei Ueshiba. It uses repetitive swinging movements in order to enhance co-ordination and mobility. These exercises are particularly effective accompanied by music with a slight beat, meaning that they're particularly good for those who are less comfortable with the 'meditative' aspects of yoga and tai chi.

especially as you grow older. It makes it easier to take full, deep breaths, and to use your back and abdominal muscles to support you. On an aesthetic level, walking taller makes you look thinner. As a guide, think of your spine as a magnetic pole. The shoulders are pulled back and down towards it, and the stomach and buttocks are also pulled in to its 'magnetic' field.

2. Stretching forces you to breathe better. If you snatch at breaths and take them from the chest instead of the diaphragm, less oxygen gets into the blood and energy levels dip. Breathing techniques have always been seen as relaxing, but now it's thought that deep breathing boosts your oxygen intake and feeds your metabolism.

Tai Chi

Tai chi was developed by the Chinese. It's very calming – sometimes called 'moving meditation' – but it requires real concentration to do it properly. Tai chi is all about beneficially directing the body's flow of energy through a series of slow movements that concentrate on balance and breathing. It is a good class if you want to relax and improve concentration, but it will not have a profound effect on your body shape. (Water tai chi, a new variation, will do this better.) Regular practice has also been shown to improve mild high blood pressure, asthma and arthritis. Qigong, another ancient Chinese system, requires less concentration. This discipline involves assimilating your internal and external chi, through slow, deliberate movements and meditation. Movements are larger and more sweeping, meaning your muscles get more of a workout.

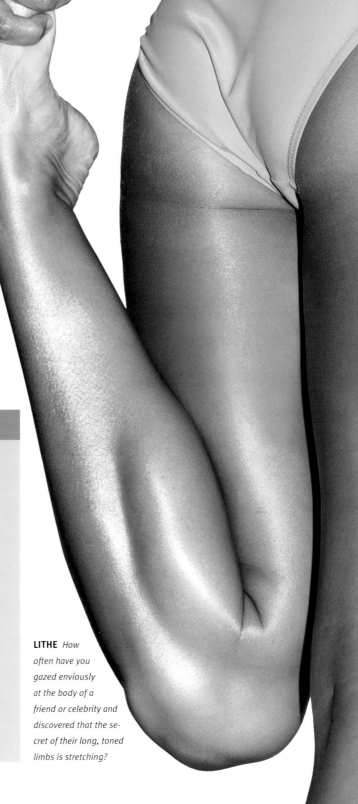

LITHE *How often have you gazed enviously at the body of a friend or celebrity and discovered that the secret of their long, toned limbs is stretching?*

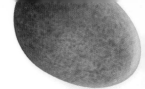

look and feel good

The growing interest in the 'internal' aspects of our bodies – what we put into them and how we keep them fit – has led to a new shift in our attitudes towards how they look on the outside, too. Meet the new wellbeing treatments.

INSIDE AND OUT

Once the idea was that beauty treatments were totally distinct from health procedures, whereas now the two worlds of health and beauty are merging, as we begin to realise that what makes us feel good on the inside will reflect how we appear on the outside.

At the heart of this transformation is a new kind of beauty phenomenon: the spa. A far cry from the pink, fluffy beauty 'salons' of yore, spas are more likely to be low-key, relaxing, gender-neutral and based around natural ingredients and therapies, focusing as much on spiritual wellbeing as outward pampering.

If you've never visited a spa, the prospect can be quite daunting. You will probably be confronted with a long list of treatments and be expected to choose one based on very little information. First, you should think about what you want to achieve. Are you looking for a relaxing treatment or an invigorating one? Perhaps your mood is not an issue, and you are simply visiting the spa to sort your skin out – for example to slough away your dry, flaky winter skin and leave you ready for those flesh-baring skimpy summer dresses. This explanation of the latest body treatments should help you decide. But whatever you go for in the end, remember that the essence of a good spa treatment is to leave you feeling as good inside as you look on the outside.

WELLBEING TREATMENTS

MASSAGE is usually a full-body treatment, although you can often get a neck, back and shoulders-only variety if you're not comfortable with baring all. Firm strokes soothe and relax aching muscles. Massage is good for feelings of fatigue and stress, sluggish circulation or bad posture. An aromatherapy massage is pretty much the same as a regular massage, but your therapist will use essential oils tailored to your needs – for example, lavender or sandalwood to relax, rosemary or lemon to invigorate. This type of massage is good for the times when you'd like to address a particular mental state as well as a physical one – for example, tiredness, lack of concentration, or inability to wind down. Finally, a deep tissue massage uses stronger pressure than normal. The idea is to penetrate deep enough beneath the skin's surface to be able to soothe aching muscles – this is particularly good for sporty types and those who like a firm-pressure massage.

During a course of Thai massage, your therapist will bend your limbs into various positions in order to be able to thoroughly penetrate all the muscles – particularly those that carry the most pressure, for example, beneath the shoulder blades. This kind of treatment isn't for everyone, but is well worth considering if you put stress on your body through strenuous workouts or sports.

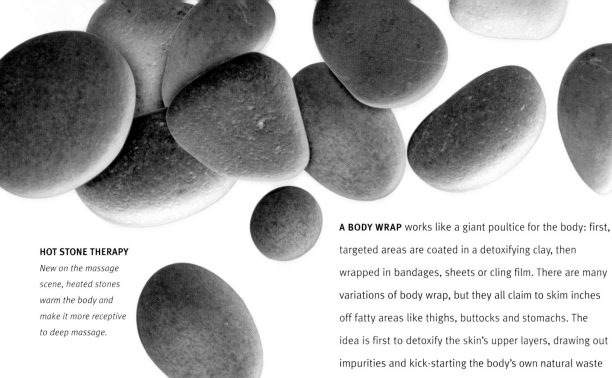

HOT STONE THERAPY

*New on the massage
scene, heated stones
warm the body and
make it more receptive
to deep massage.*

HOT STONE THERAPY is a recently devised treatment that involves small, smooth rocks that are heated and then placed beneath your back and along your arms and legs. The rocks used in this treatment are volcanic, meaning that they retain their heat, warming your body tissue so that it's more 'pliable' and receptive to massage. A perfect way to relax your body and your mind.

BEAUTY TREATMENTS

A BODY POLISH is a full-body exfoliation. Although they're not as relaxing as a straightforward massage, most body polishes start with a body scrub and then end with a moisturising body cream or oil being massaged into the skin. They can be blissfully relaxing, and also slough away dead cells to leave your skin refreshed, rehydrated and positively glowing.

A BODY WRAP works like a giant poultice for the body: first, targeted areas are coated in a detoxifying clay, then wrapped in bandages, sheets or cling film. There are many variations of body wrap, but they all claim to skim inches off fatty areas like thighs, buttocks and stomachs. The idea is first to detoxify the skin's upper layers, drawing out impurities and kick-starting the body's own natural waste disposal system and second, to compress the soft fatty tissues so that skin appears smoother and firmer. Sometimes the detoxifying products are applied ice-cool, boosting circulation and making the toxin elimination process even more efficient. Don't expect this to be relaxing – the freezing body packs make an already fairly disquieting experience distinctly uncomfortable!

LYMPHATIC DRAINAGE is the ultimate detoxifying treatment. Essentially a light massage, it is a powerful way to ease water retention and toxin build-up, and works by stimulating the lymph system. Often used in the treatment of cellulite, it's so gentle that it can also be performed after surgery to aid the healing of scars. One of its unique properties is its ability to transform the nervous system from its 'daytime' (sympathetic) state to its 'night-time' (parasympathetic) state, encouraging the body to undertake the kind of regenerative work normally reserved for when we are asleep.

BODY BEAUTIFUL

There's nothing nicer than lavishing a delicious, scented product on your skin. But how can you choose between the vast array of textures and technologies now available?

CHOOSE BETTER SKIN

If you want a satin-soft, super-smooth body, scrubs are best. Natural options include salts, sugars, crushed nuts and seeds, which are nourishing but must be applied with caution – the jagged shapes can sometimes scratch the skin. The newer, synthetic options are best for delicate skins as they're perfectly spherical. Just skim lightly across the skin's surface once or twice a week. Remember that the dead skin cells are loosened only as you rinse off, so spend plenty of time splashing water on your skin afterwards.

If your priority is to get your skin seriously clean, soaps and foaming gels can feel fabulous but will leave the skin dry and even irritated. The new varieties with their exceptional lathering qualities that claim to be better at cleansing are usually not much different to the old ones – you simply have to rinse for longer to wash them off, making you feel extra clean. Clays, on the other hand, are excellent deep-cleansers, and can act like 'face masks' for your body, drawing out impurities and firming the skin's surface. The best time to apply a clay is after exfoliating. Smooth a thin layer of clay onto clean skin and allow to dry – it usually takes about fifteen minutes. Wash off with a muslin cloth, using small, circular movements and plenty of warm water.

Special body sprays and gels claim to tighten up the skin's surface, but dry skin brushing (without products) is generally agreed to be the most effective way of achieving firm and fabulous skin. It's a daily commitment, but you'll see results in days. Take a brush with natural bristles and, starting at your feet and working upwards, brush your skin using long, sweeping upward movements (always brush towards your heart). Always brush dry skin – the ideal time would be just before you jump into a bath or shower. It'll feel a bit painful at first, but after a few days your skin will get used to it and you'll begin to love the tingling feeling.

Home spa

✳ **THE** true 'spa' experience isn't about super-swanky products, it's about creating a feeling of deep relaxation and cleanliness. For the ultimate body-unwinder, set aside a few hours and follow our simple five-step plan:

1. Prepare Switch your answer machine on, light a candle and shut the bathroom door. Make sure you have every product you're going to need with you before you start.

2. Relax Run a bath and add a relaxing bath product. Lavender and bergamot essential oils are especially good. Listen to some music if that helps – it will be most relaxing if it's something you know really well.

3. Cleanse Create a beauty 'ritual', applying an exfoliator followed by a cleansing mask.

4. Unwind After your bath, don't leap straight into your clothes. Wrap yourself in fluffy warm towels – maintaining a warm body temperature will help you to stay relaxed.

5. Soothe Before you dress, smother your body in a rich cream or oil to trap in all the goodness and moisture from your bath. Don't apply products while your skin is still wet – the water will simply dilute them – but don't leave it too long, or you'll be losing out on that essential moisture. About 5–10 minutes afterwards is perfect.

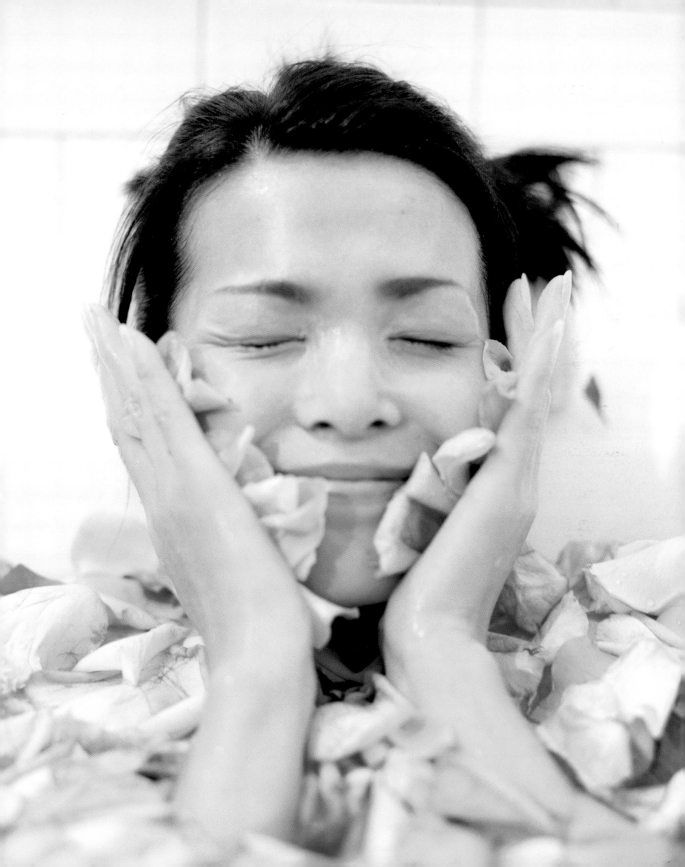

surgery: what, when, how

Cosmetic surgery used to be taboo, but these days, that's all changed. Now, the biggest problem is sorting through the abundance of alternatives and, when you've decided what you'd like, knowing the right way to go about it. The crucial thing is not to remain in the dark – so arm yourself with these vital facts first.

WHICH PROCEDURE?

For most women, deciding what to have done isn't a problem. However, advancing technology may mean there's a less drastic solution to your problem – for example, a breast lift (where the nipple and tissue are repositioned) instead of breast augmentation (where implants are inserted). If you're as specific as possible when it comes to telling your surgeon what you want to achieve, you should be told of any new procedures that might be worth considering.

Factors such as your age, health, condition of your skin and your existing features and healing patterns all impact on results, so always be honest. Smoking is a particularly big issue. Nicotine and carbon monoxide (both found in tobacco) inhibit the wound-healing process and increase the risk of pulmonary complications to such an extent that many surgeons insist that you quit smoking at least two weeks (ideally earlier) before all invasive surgical procedures, particularly breast reduction, tummy tucks and face-lifts.

TAKING THE PLUNGE

Contrary to popular belief, not all cosmetic work lasts forever. Of course, nose reshaping and lipoplasty both have permanent (and irreversible) effects, but procedures that involve stretching skin – brow lifts, face-lifts, lip lifts and buttock lifts, for example, have a 'shelf life' – gravity ensures that sagging skin is an inevitable part of growing old. These operations will usually last around ten years, although the younger you have them done, the better. A face-lift at forty – the minimum age required by most surgeons – will 'hold' for about ten years, whereas a lift at fifty will last for only six or seven.

The timing of your operation could also be important. For example, abdominoplasty (tummy tuck) has one of the most painful post-operation periods, so you'll need to find a time when you can take two or three weeks off work. If you're a hay fever sufferer, you'll need to avoid nose reshaping operations in high season, as sneezing will be a problem. In terms of your monthly cycle, your pain threshold is lowest in the week leading up to your period – try to schedule any operations for after your period instead.

SELECTING A SURGEON

Finding the right surgeon is the single most important part of the procedure. In the UK, any doctor can call himself a 'plastic' or 'cosmetic' surgeon and legally perform cosmetic operations, so before you even consider an appointment, make sure you find someone who is an accredited plastic surgeon (a surgeon who is on the Specialist Register for

Plastic Surgery of the General Medical Council). You can also contact the British Association of Aesthetic Plastic Surgeons or BAAPS (*see* Contacts) for information on specially trained cosmetic plastic surgeons. Even then, it's worth visiting several surgeons and finding the one you feel most comfortable with. Also, ask your GP, who will have dealings with local surgeons.

When talking to your surgeon, try to be as specific as possible about what you want to change. Don't look upon surgery as the magic answer to all your body foibles – think

'enhancing' rather than 'correcting' and your expectations will be much more realistic and positive. Be sceptical about surgeries that advertise widely on TV and in newspapers. Word of mouth is a much better recommendation.

Finally, when it comes to 'before' and 'after' photos, don't be fooled. There are tricks that surgeons can use to make their results appear extra impressive. Lighting wrinkles from the side makes them appear deeper; light in front of the face makes them less noticeable. Similarly, green-/blue-tinged light makes wrinkles show up more than yellow/red light.

Popular surgery options

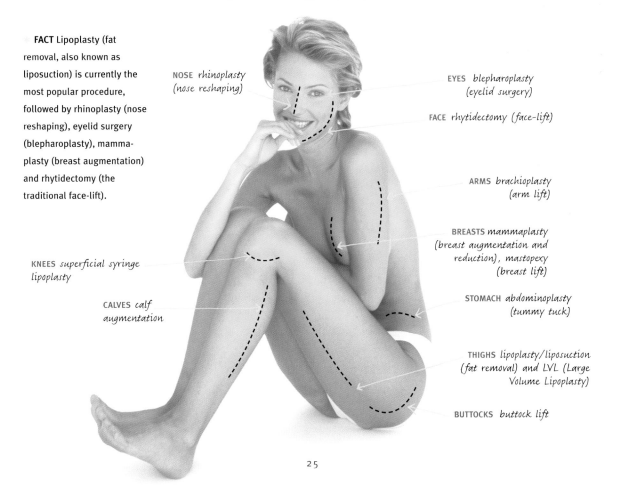

FACT Lipoplasty (fat removal, also known as liposuction) is currently the most popular procedure, followed by rhinoplasty (nose reshaping), eyelid surgery (blepharoplasty), mammaplasty (breast augmentation) and rhytidectomy (the traditional face-lift).

NOSE *rhinoplasty (nose reshaping)*

EYES *blepharoplasty (eyelid surgery)*

FACE *rhytidectomy (face-lift)*

ARMS *brachioplasty (arm lift)*

BREASTS *mammaplasty (breast augmentation and reduction), mastopexy (breast lift)*

KNEES *superficial syringe lipoplasty*

CALVES *calf augmentation*

STOMACH *abdominoplasty (tummy tuck)*

THIGHS *lipoplasty/liposuction (fat removal) and LVL (Large Volume Lipoplasty)*

BUTTOCKS *buttock lift*

SCULPT YOUR BODY

Advances in surgery mean that weight loss is no longer all about what we eat. Lipoplasty (or liposuction) is now the most popular form of cosmetic surgery, accounting for nearly half of all procedures. It provides fat removal without diet or exercise, and it targets specific fatty areas of the body, which neither diet nor exercise can do. The procedure involves injecting a saline, or salt water, solution under the skin and then inserting a long stainless steel tube (called a cannula) through a series of small incisions (less than 1 cm/ $\frac{1}{2}$ inch long) into the fat layer just beneath the skin. A vacuum pump attached to the cannula suctions away the fat cells in the selected areas. As fat is removed, the saline solution is pumped around the body to reduce blood loss – the more fat that's removed, the more liquid gets pumped in. There are a number of different techniques, most of which involve a smaller or larger volume of injected saline and the addition of lidocaine (a local anaesthetic) and/or epinephrine (to reduce bleeding). A newer technique that some doctors use employs ultrasound technology to break the walls of fat cells, releasing the fat and making it easier to suck out.

There are no hard and fast rules about how much fat you can have removed, but surgeons have always asserted that lipoplasty works best for body sculpting (shaping

Lipo info

LIPOPLASTY works wonders on hard-to-shift fat around the hips and thighs, but know all the facts before you take the plunge.

1. Lipoplasty is a speciality. Ask your surgeon how often he or she performs the procedure, and ask to see before and after photographs of cases operated on by the chosen surgeon.

2. Lipoplasty often involves follow-up procedures. Ask your surgeon what the policy is for revisions – you may find yourself paying extra for things like removal of stitches.

3. Lipoplasty doesn't get rid of cellulite – some non-medical practitioners claim endermology gets better results, though they are temporary. This is a system of rolling the skin and applying a vacuum externally at the same time.

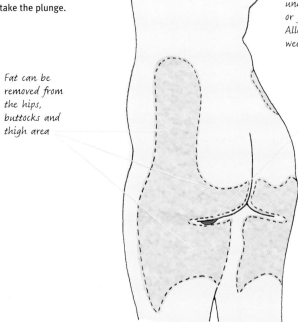

Operation is performed under a local, regional or general anaesthetic. Allow at least two weeks for recovery

Fat can be removed from the hips, buttocks and thigh area

A cannula (a long hollow metal tube) is inserted through a small incision in skin, usually hidden in the gluteal crease. Fat is sucked out of fat pockets by a vacuum instrument

thighs or trimming the waist) rather than serious weight reduction (taking you down three or four dress sizes). Localised fat areas, such as 'saddle bags' on thighs, 'love handles' at the waist or disproportionately large hips are prime areas for lipoplasty because they are often stubbornly resistant to diet and exercise. Lipoplasty can also be combined with abdominoplasty (tummy tuck). Smaller fat deposits, for example around the knees or ankles, can also be removed, but this is normally done with a syringe.

It's inadvisable to use lipoplasty as a way to jump-start a weight-loss programme. If you want to lose weight, it's best to go on a diet before the surgery. In general, lipoplasty is intended for people who are close to normal weight (no more than 30 per cent over their ideal body weight). Recently, however, some surgeons have been performing what is termed large-volume lipoplasty (LVL), which uses the ultrasound-assisted technique to remove 5 litres ($10\frac{1}{2}$ pints) of fat aspirate (about 10 lbs/4.5 kilos) or more in one session and can be done on people who are up to 50 lbs (22.6 kilos) overweight. To qualify for this kind of surgery, you must be in excellent health. Eating disorders, weight fluctuation of more than 10 lbs (4.5 kilos) within the past year, alcoholism and drug abuse prohibit the operation.

BEFORE

Before the operation, be sure to discuss with the doctor how you should prepare yourself, including what you should or should not eat or drink, and whether you should stop taking certain medications such as aspirin. If you are a smoker, you will be instructed to stop smoking in advance of the surgery. Ask questions so you will have a realistic idea of

what the procedure and the aftermath will be like, and what you can expect during the healing period. You will probably want to arrange to have someone take you home afterwards.

DURING

Lipoplasty is done under local, regional or general anaesthesia, and during an operation, you can have more than one area of fat removed at a time. Operations last for anywhere between one and four hours. The procedure is not without its risks: some are potentially life-threatening and include infection, allergic reactions, toxic shock, potentially severe burns, embolisms (blood clots that can damage vital organs), severe swelling, compression of nerves, abnormal heart rhythms and heart failure.

AFTER

For the first few days after the treatment, you may lose some blood and fluids from the affected areas. As with any major surgery, you need to leave a good couple of weeks' recovery time, and there are post-operative restrictions on activities such as physical exercise and flying.

The good news is that once the fat cells are gone, you'll never be fat in that area again (if you do gain weight, the fat will simply settle somewhere else). In the future, surgeons predict that lipoplasty will become even less painful and even more high-tech. Computer-assisted surgery is a possibility, giving surgeons greater accuracy – which will be particularly good for smaller fat deposits. Work is also being done to assess whether fat removed by lipoplasty can be engineered for reuse elsewhere in the same body – for example, in reconstructive surgery and breast augmentation.

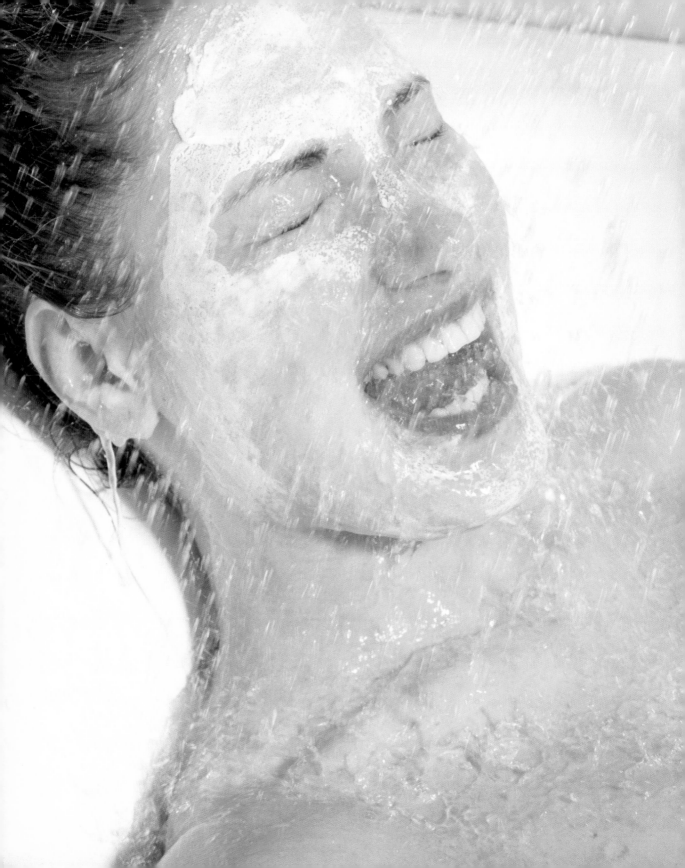

top

We've discussed the body in general, now let's take it from the top with the part of your body that is seen the most by people. It's no wonder that so many of the everyday phrases we use include the face: we face the future, face forward, face up to things and face facts. In short, your face is always on show, and as you project it to the outside world, so it acts as a barometer for your health and wellbeing. Or does it? New treatments in facial surgery, along with fabulous new beauty treatments, mean that you can accentuate, enhance or disguise virtually any of your features. Similarly, new techniques for your teeth, hair and eyes mean there's now no reason for you never to look truly groomed. Add to this the latest thinking on how your diet and lifestyle affects your skin, plus facial exercises to turn back time, and soon you'll be facing the world with a fabulous new look.

healthy skin deep down
Beauty isn't skin deep. No matter how much faith we put in the latest lotions and potions, there'll always be something that beauty products can't achieve: a firm foundation for the face that comes from the state of our health beneath the skin's surface. While products can smooth, moisturise and refine the skin's upper layers, truly healthy-looking skin can be achieved only by cosseting from within, with a daily dose of the right vitamins and nutrients.

GOOD SKIN FROM WITHIN

Often we're so despondent about the state of our skin that we don't know where to start, but when it comes to solving deep-rooted skin problems, a targeted approach is always best. Choose the part that you'd most like to work on, and discover how to serve up a gorgeous complexion.

PLUMP, FIRM AND HYDRATED

Healthy skin equals plump skin – anything less can leave you looking haggard. The essential fatty acids (EFAs) are important allies when it comes to skin health. They play a huge role in the immune system and are vital for the formation of cells. Skin marred by dry, greyish patches is a sign of a diet poor in EFAs. These are the 'good fats' and you can get them only from food. To be sure that you're getting enough EFAs, include some of the following in your diet: oily fish such as mackerel, herring, sardines, fresh tuna, trout and salmon; nuts, sunflower seeds and sunflower oil. Vitamin A also helps to keep the skin's natural oils (sebum) replenished, and too little can result in blocked pores, rough skin and acne. Vitamin A-rich foods include sesame oil, carrots, mangoes and other brightly coloured fruits, melons and tomatoes.

Two minerals that may help skin retain a youthful glow are zinc and selenium. You need only a small amount of each, so try to get it from the food you eat. Good sources of zinc are shellfish (especially oysters), red meat and poultry, whole grains, pulses and nuts. By far the best source of selenium is brazil nuts, but you can also find it in tuna and other fish, poultry, liver, and enriched pasta and bread products.

PEACHY *Fruit is rich in skin-boosting nutrients. Peaches and apricots contain beta-carotene for plump, hydrated skin. Pears also contain useful amounts of vitamin A and C.*

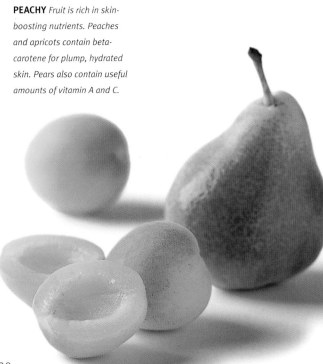

Dermatologists are often sceptical about just how much the skin can benefit from drinking copious amounts of water. You can drink a lot of water, but if it doesn't get to and stay in your skin cells, your skin will look and feel dry. Drinking water is key, but so is keeping it sealed in. Vitamin E is particularly good at that, and unlike many vitamins is equally effective when applied topically – for an instant boost for dry skin, simply burst a vitamin E capsule and massage straight into skin. Vitamin B3 (niacin) also has excellent moisture-retaining capabilities, and is found in fish, whole grains, peanuts and peas.

ILLUMINATED COLOUR

If it's that radiant, lit-from-within glow you crave, look no further than vitamin C. Its capillary-strengthening abilities mean that it helps transport nutrients to the skin's upper layers, fighting the appearance of tiny spider veins and rosacea and ensuring that the blood supply stays close to the skin's surface, giving skin a pink, rosy bloom. Vitamin C can be found in citrus fruits, guavas, kiwis, mangoes, papayas, peaches and strawberries. Antioxidants are also excellent for improving microcirculation: one super-refreshing way to get them is from green and white tea.

Top 10 anti-ageing foods

DON'T think you need to spend a fortune on expensive face creams to get plump, firm and hydrated skin. Including the following skin boosters and free-radical fighters in your diet will help you win the war against ageing. The most effective fighters are the antioxidants: vitamins A (beta-carotene), C and E, and polyphenols and flavonoids (found in tea and citrus fruits).

Food	Contains	Good for
Avocado	Vitamin E	Hydrating skin
Berries	Vitamin C	Fighting free radicals
Papaya	Vitamin C	Fighting free radicals
Carrots	Beta-carotene, zinc	Firm complexion, fighting free radicals
Citrus fruits	Vitamin C	Radiance-boosting
Purple grapes	Polyphenols	Cell renewal, fighting free radicals
Onions and garlic	Selenium, vitamin C	Boosting immune system, circulation
Spinach	Beta-carotene, folic acid, vitamin E, iron	Boosting circulation, hydrating
Tomatoes	Beta-carotene, zinc, vitamin B3	Retaining moisture
Chickpeas	Folic acid	Firm complexion, fighting free radicals, hydrating

face facts

We've all heard of facial exercises, but most of us remain sceptical. Aside from the question of what they can actually achieve, there's also the fact that most of them make you look pretty ridiculous while you're doing them. There's also a rumour that performing facial exercises can actually stretch the skin, making you look saggier than you did before. Maybe it's time to face facts and find out the real story.

WHY DO FACIAL EXERCISES?

In a market that's already saturated with creams, supplements and surgical procedures, aren't facial exercises just another way for people to cash in on our anti-ageing anxieties? Not at all. The ten muscle groups in our scalp and face are barely used to capacity, so they're relatively weak, meaning that the skin they support is prey to the effects of gravity – in other words, sagging. Also, well-exercised facial muscles pump up to ten times more blood to the skin's surface than 'untrained' ones, delivering vital oxygen and nutrients into the skin and improving its radiance and colour. Finally – and this is the one everyone likes best – facial exercise, done properly, can increase the size and strength of the underlying muscles. By increasing this muscle mass, the epidermis (skin's upper layer) stretches itself in order to accommodate this newly enlarged area of muscle. Like a creased fabric pulled taut, the act of stretching the skin effectively 'irons out' wrinkles.

WHAT CAN YOU ACHIEVE?

What you can achieve from facial exercises depends, of course, on how much effort you put in. Doing facial routines for between five and ten minutes every day should be enough for you to see results within a matter of a few weeks, although you should start to see an improvement in the general tone of your skin in less than a week. Interestingly, unlike some forms of exercise where the people who are in most need of toning up take longest to see results, facial exercises seem to produce the biggest initial improvements in those with the saggiest skin. Facial exercises are particularly useful for sun-damaged skin that has prematurely aged. However, they will never eliminate lines completely, and it's better to start young and keep exercising.

The best results from facial exercises are in the general surface of the skin. The texture can become firmer, the colour brighter and the lines diminished. Anecdotal evidence has also told of women noticing an improvement in the appearance of dark, sunken eyes, downturned creases around the lips, and forehead lines and crow's feet. It's worth mentioning here the difference between ageing lines and expression lines. When it comes to facial exercising, there isn't a distinction. Both are essentially created as a result of the effects of gravity on ageing skin, and contrary to popular belief, moving your face more, not less, is the answer to eliminating them. This is because you are increasing the muscle mass beneath the surface, gradually stretching the skin in a natural way.

Major muscle groups of the face and neck

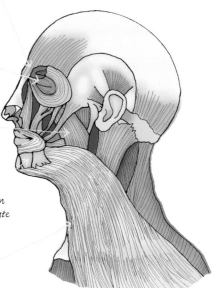

FOREHEAD MUSCLE *(occipito frontalis)* –
*exercising this muscle may
reduce frown lines.*

EYELID MUSCLES
*levator palpebra (to open
the eye) and the orbicularis
oculi (to close the eye).
Exercising these will help
reduce fine lines and bags.*

CHEEK MUSCLES *the principal muscle
is the buccinator. Working
these muscles can firm cheek area
and lift sagging jowls.*

MOUTH MUSCLES *orbicularis oris
surrounds the lip, and eleven muscles in
all are used to move the mouth. Eliminate
lip lines and creases with exercise.*

NECK MUSCLES *platysma muscles –
exercise can help firm the lax muscles
that contribute to a flabby neck.*

FACIAL exercises can help to strengthen and lift facial muscles in women of all ages. Many women report that regular facial exercise improves the skin's tone and texture, and helps to reduce the appearance of bags, fine lines and wrinkles.

It is this increase in muscle that makes facial exercising so much more effective in the long term than a face-lift. With a face-lift, the facial muscles are shortened and the skin is pulled tight. But without firming the muscles, the skin – though tighter – will inevitably sag again in time. This is why so many women have repeated face-lifts. The good news is that it's possible – in fact advisable – to do facial exercises both before and after (although obviously not immediately after) a face-lift.

For those women who are seriously concerned with facial sagging, this double whammy of a face-lift together with regular exercises is probably the way to go. For most of us, however, it's the 'regular exercise' part that we should really latch on to most. If we combine the facial exercises with anything, it should be good-quality, hydrating, skin-strengthening products. Maintaining a healthy skin structure at the dermal (deeper) level by buoying the skin's collagen and elastin levels will render skin more able to accommodate our firmed-up and newly enlarged facial muscles as they expand. Look for face creams that are specifically targeted for 'anti-ageing' and smooth generously onto face and throat.

NOW YOU TRY

These facial exercises will lift, firm, revive and re-energise your skin. Start with clean skin, clean hands, hair tied back and no rings or earrings to get in the way.

1. Skin alert FACE TAPPING

Using brisk movements, take your middle two fingers and tap the ends up the bridge of your nose and along the top of your eyebrows, then from the centre of your chin along your jaw line, and finally make circles on your cheeks. **REPEAT** all three for one minute.

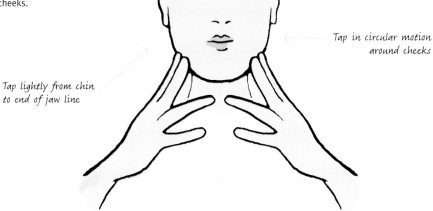

Tap lightly up the nose and along eyebrows

Tap in circular motion around cheeks

Tap lightly from chin to end of jaw line

2. Surprised (but still asleep)
EYE FIRMING

With your eyes closed, lift your eyebrows up (as if surprised) but keep your eyelids shut. Hold for a count of five, then release. **REPEAT** for thirty seconds.

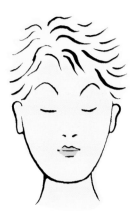

3. Inquisitive
EYE REJUVENATING

Keep your eyes open, looking straight ahead. Now look up for a count of one, then down for a count of one. **REPEAT for thirty seconds, then do the same thing going left to right, again for thirty seconds.**

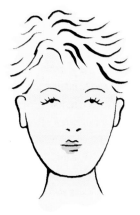

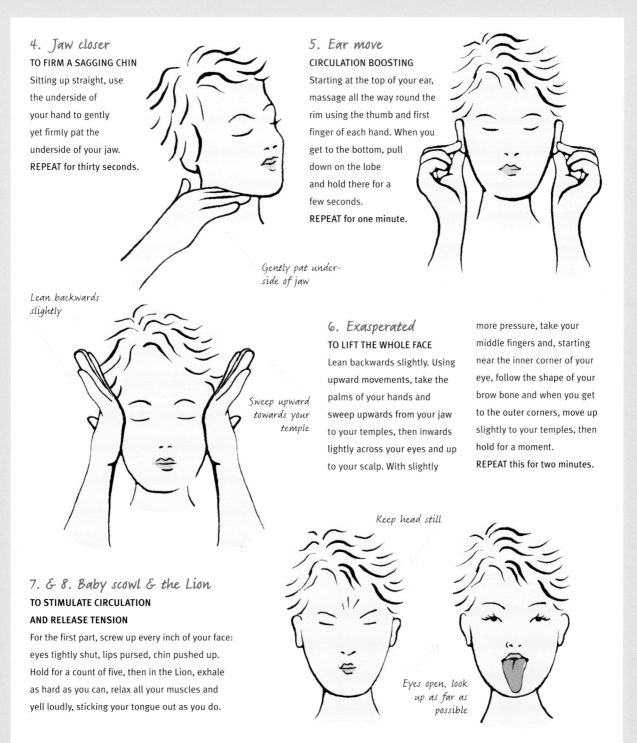

4. Jaw closer
TO FIRM A SAGGING CHIN
Sitting up straight, use
the underside of
your hand to gently
yet firmly pat the
underside of your jaw.
REPEAT for thirty seconds.

5. Ear move
CIRCULATION BOOSTING
Starting at the top of your ear,
massage all the way round the
rim using the thumb and first
finger of each hand. When you
get to the bottom, pull
down on the lobe
and hold there for a
few seconds.
REPEAT for one minute.

*Gently pat under-
side of jaw*

*Lean backwards
slightly*

*Sweep upward
towards your
temple*

6. Exasperated
TO LIFT THE WHOLE FACE
Lean backwards slightly. Using
upward movements, take the
palms of your hands and
sweep upwards from your jaw
to your temples, then inwards
lightly across your eyes and up
to your scalp. With slightly

more pressure, take your
middle fingers and, starting
near the inner corner of your
eye, follow the shape of your
brow bone and when you get
to the outer corners, move up
slightly to your temples, then
hold for a moment.
REPEAT this for two minutes.

Keep head still

7. & 8. Baby scowl & the Lion
**TO STIMULATE CIRCULATION
AND RELEASE TENSION**
For the first part, screw up every inch of your face:
eyes tightly shut, lips pursed, chin pushed up.
Hold for a count of five, then in the Lion, exhale
as hard as you can, relax all your muscles and
yell loudly, sticking your tongue out as you do.

*Eyes open, look
up as far as
possible*

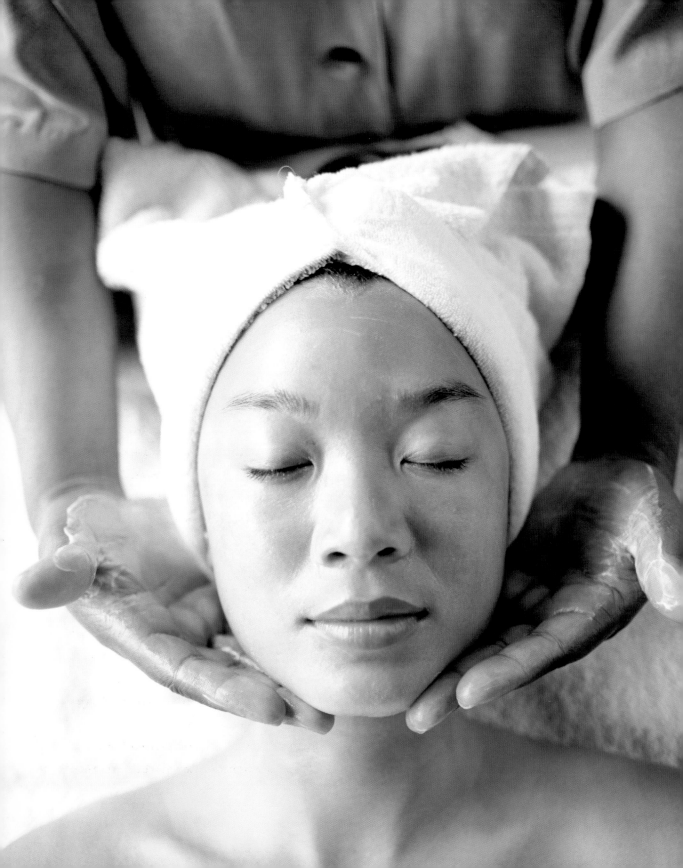

clean and serene

So you've decided to book in for a facial. What can you expect from a treatment, and, more important, what can you achieve? Being touched on the face is a wonderfully relaxing, yet highly intimate procedure, so you need to know that you're in good hands. Before you take the plunge, here are the facial facts you should know.

WHAT CAN YOU EXPECT?

These days, salon facials aren't only about working on your face. The advent of the 'holistic' approach to skincare means that you're as likely to begin a facial with a scalp massage or a foot bath as you are with your face. Facialists say that adding on these extras helps them to remind you that your face is only one part of your whole body, so that it's easier to understand that what you do to your body will have a direct bearing on how you look. Sometimes you can also get added beautifying touches such as eyebrow shaping, and another recent addition is the inclusion of a 'pick and mix' section where you'll be able to choose another area such as your back or arms to have massaged in the fifteen minutes while, for example, your face mask is getting to work.

Ordinarily, though, a facial will consist of a thorough cleanse, perhaps incorporating a machine that gently directs steam at your face; exfoliation (sometimes a scrub, a mask or a gentle peel); a hydrating mask; and then a moisturiser or facial oil. After the exfoliation you might also be offered extractions – the removal of blackheads and tiny blemishes. Be warned – these can hurt! Sometimes it helps to clench your fists at the same time – and extractions aren't a good idea if you're planning to go out straight after your treatment, as they often look red and angry for a few hours afterwards. Piling the make-up straight on might also undo some of that good work, too.

One of the hardest-working treatments is a Lymphatic Drainage facial. As we saw with lymphatic body treatments, they are particularly good for combating water retention, so choose this kind of facial if you are prone to puffiness. For out-and-out relaxation, an Indian face massage is fantastic. Based on the principles of Ayurveda, it involves massage that focuses on the third eye (middle of the forehead) to rebalance your body's energy centres. Traditional treatments can involve pouring oil directly onto this spot – so relaxing it has to be felt to be believed.

With other kind of facials, there is huge room for interpretation. One treatment often cited is the 'European Facial'. For some salons, this means a method that involves lots of circulation-boosting massage, and for others it signifies a very thorough treatment, including lots of extractions. Similarly, an 'Aromatherapy Facial' can involve anything from a personally prescribed cocktail of essential oils applied directly to your skin, to nothing more complicated than a relaxing scented candle being placed in the room during your treatment. As with any salon procedure, it's better to ask about what the name means before you book.

NON-SURGICAL FACE-LIFTS

In the same way that you can get toning tables to work the muscles on your body, you can now get machines designed to do the same for your face. Some work on the outside by attaching pads to the skin's surface, like CACI®, the original non-surgical facial procedure. CACI® has evolved since its invention so that it can now be placed on different settings according to your biggest concerns, although it's most associated with improving puffiness and sagging skin. Others, such as the ERP Face Magic system, are invasive, inserting tiny needles into the face so that they can work beneath the skin's surface. In both cases, an electromagnetic current is passed through the probes to stimulate the facial muscles.

Dibitron is one of the most space-age procedures and is particularly effective for rejuvenating acne-prone skins – you wear a helmet with electronically controlled pads inside. They are attached to your face and stimulate the facial muscles to give an effect similar to a vigorous massage. Opinion is divided as to how much difference these treatments can make over the long term, but it's fairly safe to say that they work best after a course of appointments. This can be expensive in the long run, but perhaps not when compared with the expense and upheaval of a 'real' face-lift.

BEAUTIFUL TO THE TOUCH

How your skin looks and feels is closely interrelated: if your skin is not touchably soft and silky, it won't look good, and vice versa. Similarly, having a facial is about more than just achieving beautiful, super-clean skin. Of course, that's the main aim, but a good facial should also be as relaxing as it is beautifying. Some women prefer having a facial than a back massage to relieve stress. If you're uncomfortable about getting completely undressed for a treatment, your inhibitions might prevent you from having a truly relaxing experience, so a facial might be a better choice.

AT-HOME TREATMENTS

For most of us, though, going for a facial is a once-in-a-while treat. So can you create a similar experience for yourself? Nowadays beauty companies recommend specific ways in which to massage in their products at home. Many premium brands supply instructions with each pot of face cream they sell, and mass market companies are getting in on the act, too. You can even get cleansers that have special 'rituals' to follow. They're usually in the form of a pomade (like solidified oil) that you apply directly to the skin, then 'polish' off with a hot muslin cloth. But for most modern women, the thought of having a skincare routine that involves anything more than the most cursory splash of water and quick dab of cream is optimistic to say the least. So why bother?

It's with moisturisers that at-home facials really come into their own. It makes sense to massage your moisturiser into your skin – it will help the cream sink in properly so it doesn't just sit on the surface, and it will also stimulate your circulation, helping to eliminate those radiance-sapping toxins. The most effective way to massage in your face cream is this: first, make sure your hands are super clean. Then take just a tiny bit more than your usual amount of moisturiser and rub it quickly between your hands – this will warm the cream up so it's easier to spread evenly over the whole face. Using the whole of your palms, press the cream into your cheeks and then with your fingertips, follow your orbital bone (beneath the eye socket) forwards and backwards. Don't go too near to the eye – especially if you intend to use a separate eye cream later. Then, sweep your fingers up towards your temples, continuing towards your forehead. Keep moving your hands up so that now only your palms rest on your forehead. Next, bring your hands down vertically, right to the bottom of your face, covering the forehead, nose and chin in product. Now with the tips of your fingers, trace along the jaw line, working forwards and back so that you can really feel the tissue beneath the skin's surface. The key thing to remember is that, like any good facialist, your hands should never completely leave the face until you've finished.

Even if you can't manage this every day, once or twice a week would be fantastic. For a really thorough beneath-the-surface cleanse, start off with a gentle exfoliating scrub to eliminate dead surface cells. Follow with a face mask. For deep cleansing, choose one that's designed to purify the skin. It will most likely be clay-based — clay is porous and acts like a sponge, drawing impurities to the surface as the mask dries. Washing the clay off properly afterwards is essential. Soften the layer bit by bit with warm water (cold won't dissolve the dirt), then make small circles with your fingers all over your face until the clay has disappeared. Next, spritz with toner if you use one or go straight to your moisturiser, following the massaging steps.

Facial scrubs and masks

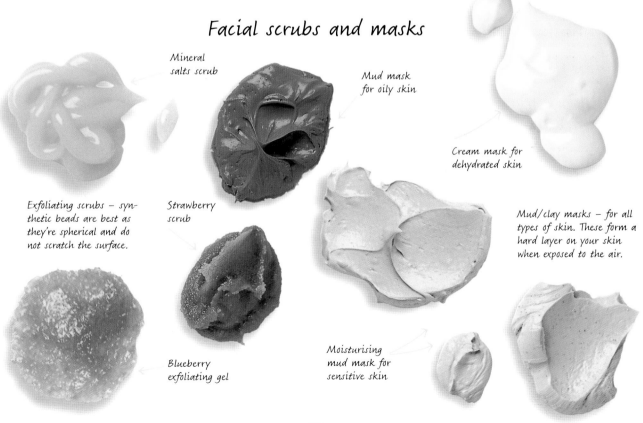

Mineral salts scrub

Mud mask for oily skin

Cream mask for dehydrated skin

Exfoliating scrubs – synthetic beads are best as they're spherical and do not scratch the surface.

Strawberry scrub

Mud/clay masks – for all types of skin. These form a hard layer on your skin when exposed to the air.

Blueberry exfoliating gel

Moisturising mud mask for sensitive skin

repair and renew With surgery, you can alter things that niggle you and boost your self-confidence into the bargain. The procedures listed here will help alter what nature gave you – or slow down the hands of time – while still achieving a 'natural' look.

REPAIR ME

Originally, cosmetic surgery involved only operations such as nose reshaping, which are designed to 'correct' or improve what nature gave us. In these days of 'lunchtime' procedures and 'conveyor belt' quick-fixes, that's all changed, but corrective surgery still forms a major part of a surgeon's workload. In these restorative operations, the changes made aren't purely superficial – surgeons need to work beneath the skin's surface, sometimes even chiselling away at bones. This means that they're among the most serious operations in the cosmetic surgery repertoire (most are performed under general anaesthetic), so they shouldn't be considered lightly. Having said that, the psychological benefits of cosmetic surgery can't be underestimated. There are countless stories of men and women who, post-surgery, have found the confidence to get a new job, meet a new partner or make dozens of tiny but empowering changes to their everyday lives.

RHINOPLASTY (NOSE RESHAPING)

There are two undisputed facts about the nose: it is our single most defining facial feature; changes to it, no matter how small, can alter the face appreciably. Too big, too small, too pointed, too flat, too crooked, too long, too narrow, too flared – the list of nasal bugbears is endless.

And for every one of those complaints, there's a knock-on effect on how its alteration will affect other parts of the face – particularly the chin, which serves to 'balance out' the nose. A small chin, for example, makes the nose appear larger and surgeons will often recommend a chin augmentation at the same time as a nasal operation. In nasal surgery, the incisions are normally made either inside the nose or on the central panel between the nostrils. The skin is lifted away from the bone, and the bone and cartilage beneath is reshaped. You'll need to wear a splint on the nose for about a week after, but bruising may last for up to a fortnight.

MENTOPLASTY (CHIN RESHAPING)

Chin reshaping can do one of two things: augment a receding chin, either by inserting synthetic implants or moving the bone forward; or diminish a too prominent chin by sculpting away at the bone. Like most implants, those placed in the chin may need replacing after several years. When considering mentoplasty, many people worry that the incision scars will be obvious. In both augmentation and reduction surgery, surgeons can gain access either through the mouth or under the chin, neither of which will ordinarily be visible. Sometimes, consultations with your surgeon will reveal that it's not really the bone structure of your chin that's the concern, but excess fat around the jaw line, causing 'jowls'. These can be removed using submental liposuction.

If you decide to have mentoplasty, you will have to wear a dressing for a few days after the operation, and will need to avoid solid food for up to a week. Swelling may take a month to disappear, but most patients go back to work after a fortnight.

OTOPLASTY (EAR SURGERY)

The problem with ears is not always that they stick out. Sometimes they droop, sometimes they are overly large but still flat to the head and sometimes they're asymmetrical. Happily, all these defects can be corrected with surgery. Ears that stick out too far (more than 2 cm/$\frac{3}{4}$ inch is normally thought to be 'too far') can be pinned back by removing skin from and repositioning cartilage behind the ear, where it joins the head. Drooping ears are corrected by creating an artificial fold at the top, helping to hold them up. In a more minor operation, a torn earlobe can be fixed either with stitches or with tissue taken from the other ear. An added bonus – earlobes are renowned for their quick healing capacity (which is why the holes in pierced ear lobes often close up when earrings aren't worn).

MALAR AUGMENTATION (CHEEK RESHAPING)

Well-shaped cheekbones, sitting high on the cheeks, add character and definition to the face. In one of the newest procedures in the facial surgery arena, squashy silicone implants that feel very like normal facial tissue can be inserted through an incision, either in the mouth or on rare occasions through the same incision made for a blepharoplasty (lower eye bag reduction). In other cases, cheekbones can be built up using a bone substitute made from coral called hydroxyapatite granules. As with other procedures, changing the cheekbones can also affect the prominence of other facial features, most particularly making an oversize nose appear smaller. The recovery time following these procedures is around a fortnight, although swelling can last longer, and may spread up towards the eyes, making wearing glasses difficult.

RENEW ME

Surgery is not all about reshaping your facial features. It can also offer subtle changes to eliminate the signs of ageing and give your face a new lease of life.

Ageing skin has many factors to contend with. First, and most irrepressible, is gravity. Its constant pull means that over the years your skin is pulled ever downwards, and even the firmest complexion will eventually start to sag. This is where cosmetic surgery can make some of its biggest contributions. The traditional rhytidectomy (face-lift) works by pulling the skin back up to where it should be, but the 'lift' comes from around the temples, leaving a creased forehead behind – often one of the biggest wrinkle offenders. Enter the forehead lift, sometimes known as a brow lift. This literally starts at the top; incisions are made inside the hair line and the skin is pulled back so that lines and wrinkles are smoothed out and brows are prominent again. A major advantage is that with a brow lift, surgeons can target horizontal expression lines and those deeper, vertical wrinkles that sometimes appear at the top of the nose.

Many women opt for more specific 'lifts' such as this because whole face-lifts can sometimes leave patients with an odd, 'stretched' look. Because of advances in technology and surgery, it is now common practice to sculpt the tissue beneath the skin instead of just altering the surface, so that the pulled-up skin is a much better 'fit'. This is called an SMAS (superficial muscular and aponeurotic system) lift.

YOUNG EYES

The biggest advances in surgery are usually made in areas where people have expressed most concern – so it's no surprise that eye surgery is particularly advanced. We rely on our eyes to provide most of our facial expression, so when the eyelids begin to sag, we can start to look old beyond our years. Blepharoplasty (eyelid surgery) is the catch-all procedure to sort out drab-looking eyes and make them – and us – sparkle again. Small wonder that it's now become such a popular cosmetic surgery procedure for women.

The first part of the procedure happens above the eye: muscle and fat are removed through an incision in the crease of the eyelid (it's the best-hidden place on the eye) and then the overlying skin is cut back to create a tighter finish. Fat around the eyes puts extra pressure on the skin tissue, causing it to bulge and creating permanently puffy 'bags' beneath the eyes, so the second part of the procedure involves making tiny incisions in the lower lash line and removing and/or repositioning the excess fatty tissue. The whole operation usually takes less than three hours, but is longer when – as frequently happens – it is combined with a brow lift.

SENSUAL LIPS

Finally, it is possible to restore lips to their former glory, too. Drooping, 'sadness' lines that turn down the corners of the mouth can be raised by cutting out the excess skin in a lip lift. Thinning of the lips is another problem. Ageing, smoking or even just having an expressive, talkative nature are all factors that can cause lips to appear thinner as we age. Implants such as collagen or the newer synthetic varieties are a simple way to restore their fullness, but last only for around three to six months at a time.

For a more permanent lip-plumping solution, a lip augmentation can involve either taking fat from the deeper layers of the skin (a dermal fat graft) or harvesting fat cells through liposuction from another part of the patient's body, then washing it and injecting it into the lips (micro fat grafting). This can have corrective benefits as well as age-defying ones, because many people have differently proportioned lips (the upper lip is usually thinner). Also by 'plumping up' the tiny age lines that filter off the mouth, injections can stop the lipstick 'bleed' that tends to increase as we age.

Below the mouth, the buccal fat pads are those prominent fatty deposits that are found above the jaw line near the corner of the mouth. These can be removed to give a smoother look to the lower half of the face.

SMOOTH NECK

The throat is a much-neglected but oft-maligned area. For this, platysma tightening involves refirming the muscle responsible for keeping the neck and jaw line looking tight and taut. It is often performed as part of a face-lift.

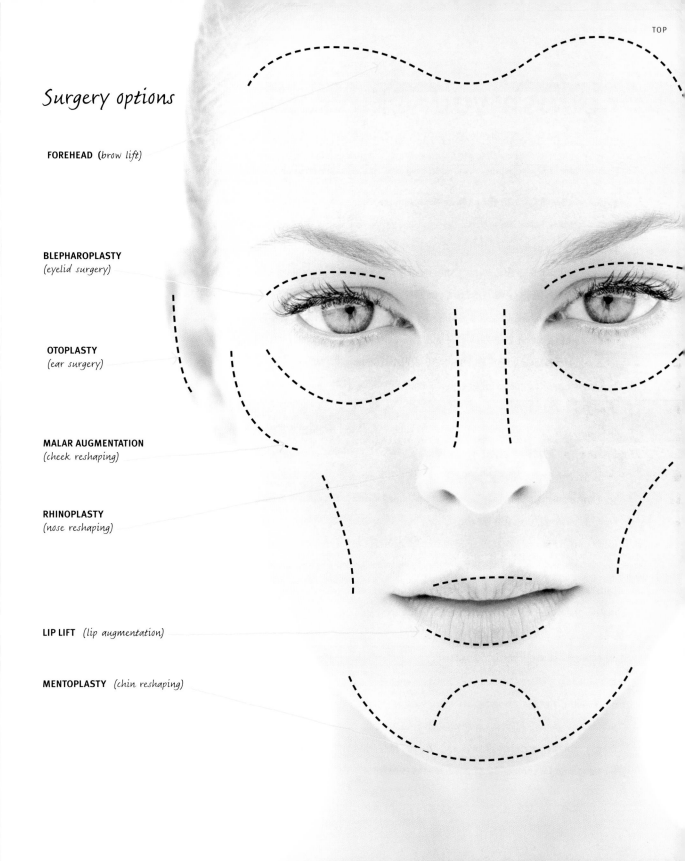

Surgery options

FOREHEAD (*brow lift*)

BLEPHAROPLASTY
(*eyelid surgery*)

OTOPLASTY
(*ear surgery*)

MALAR AUGMENTATION
(*cheek reshaping*)

RHINOPLASTY
(*nose reshaping*)

LIP LIFT (*lip augmentation*)

MENTOPLASTY (*chin reshaping*)

the workout you don't need

Regular exercise may do wonders for the body, but it can also play havoc with the skin. You've worked hard to get a toned, fit body, so don't ruin it by neglecting your skincare routine. Here's how to avoid the perils of a fitness freak's complexion.

INDOORS

Let's start with the gym. The key word for skin at any time is hydration, but when it comes to aerobic exercise in a hot, stuffy environment such as a gym, drinking an adequate supply of water is not so much a matter of comfort as a matter of urgency. Without vigorous exercise, you normally lose about 2 liters ($4\frac{1}{4}$ pints) of water a day, only some of it through perspiration. Adding a good sweaty session at the gym will significantly increase the volume lost.

When you are dehydrated, the blood flow to your skin is reduced, and over time this can result in a kind of grey pallor. In the long term, you'll also find that the diminishing number of nutrients reaching the skin affects its daily renewal process, meaning skin can become dry and flaky, and washing several times a day will only exacerbate this. Hardly surprising, the best way to combat these effects – not only for your skin but also for your general fitness performance – is to drink more water. Drink 500 ml (1 pint) of water around two hours before exercise, then 250 ml ($\frac{1}{2}$ pint) when you arrive at the gym – and around every fifteen minutes during your workout. If the thought of this makes you queasy during exercise, chances are you're already dehydrated. Gym skin also needs extra care on the outside. Exfoliate with a gentle body scrub at least two or three times a week and apply body lotion after showering.

Swimming indoors also brings its own perils. Chlorinated pools leave skin dry, dry, dry – and also leave that lingering 'detergent' smell, so it's vital to wash straight after a dip. Use a highly lathering shower gel (the lather doesn't make you cleaner, but the extra time it takes to wash off means your body's getting drenched with extra water) and apply it twice, rinsing in between, in the same way that you would a shampoo on your hair. Again, body lotion afterwards is a must, but keep chemical fragrances to a minimum – they can add to skin dryness.

OUTDOORS

With all those indoor perils, it may seem as if a run or jog outside in the fresh air would be the perfect way to improve your body and skin together. Oxygen certainly does wonders for radiance-boosting, but there are still some factors to be aware of. If you're jogging in the city, for example, your skin is exposed to pollution, and wherever you're exercising there's always the question of those wrinkle-inducing UV rays. Fine, you might think, I'll just wear an SPF lotion while I run. The problem is that not all skin creams are alike. An SPF is good (factor 15–30 depending on the sun strength and time of day), but make sure you don't use a wax-based formulation. The pores on the face are tiny, and these thick, heavy sun protection creams can be comedogenic (pore-clogging), especially when mixed with perspiration. It's also important to wash your face properly after outdoor exercise. Perspiration mingles with sebum and forms a substance that attracts dirt, and if you don't wash it away, it will literally sit there all day.

No matter how much water you drink, perspiration is a normal part of exercise – even on the face. Keep your facial temperature low by drinking plenty of water, and try a facial mist, too. Also, if you've drunk more than a glass or two of alcohol in the evening, don't exercise the following morning – you'll sweat much more than you would normally.

Another pore-clogging peril is make-up, but there's one simple make-up rule when it comes to exercising: don't wear any. Not only will it run as you start to perspire (and mascara halfway down your cheeks is not a good look) but the rise in temperature will help it work its way further down into your pores, making it even harder to clean off afterwards. If you can't bear to face the world without even a smattering of colour, look for mineral-based make-ups that are non-comedogenic and won't run, and a water- or gel-based foundation. And as in most situations in life, a little bit of lipstick won't do any harm!

SWEATY BETTY *When it comes to workouts, water is a must both internally and externally. Drink plenty of water before and during exercise, and always cleanse your skin thoroughly afterwards to get rid of pore-clogging perspiration.*

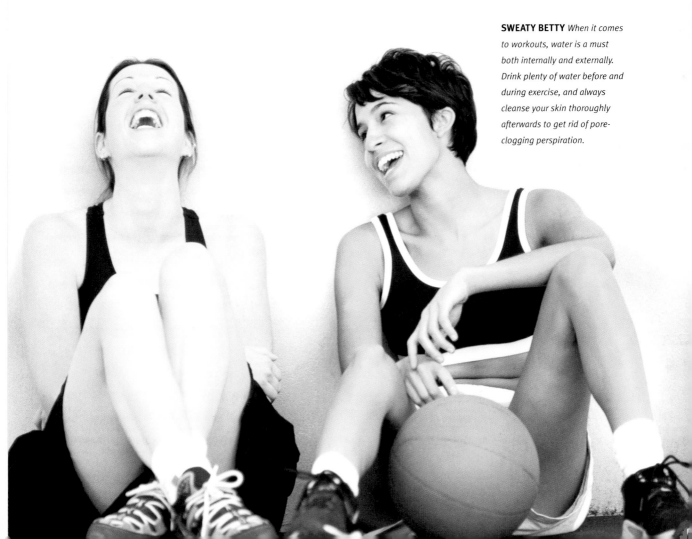

MODERN SKIN

Wander around any beauty hall and you'd be forgiven for thinking that there are as many creams and lotions on offer as there are faces in the world to put them on. All that choice can be bewildering, but if you get to know a few key ingredients and how they work, you can find the product that will work hardest for you.

AHAS There's now an AHA version of nearly every skincare product you can buy. The abbreviation stands for alpha hydroxy acids, although companies wishing to sound a little more natural often call them fruit acids (some are derived from foods such as apples and grapes). Their basic advantage is that they can exfoliate the skin's superficial layers to reveal a smooth new layer underneath. While it may seem that this would be gentler than, say, using a grainy scrub to do the same job, it's important not to over-load your skin with these acids – especially if your skin is young or sensitive. Check labels and beware of using more than one AHA product a day because experts believe this will be too much for your skin.

ANTIOXIDANTS These are beauty's stress-busters – vitamins such as A (beta-carotene), C and E that help to fight the toxins in the skin caused by stress, pollution, cigarette smoke and even UV rays. Recent scientific research also shows that a healthy dose of antioxidants can effectively reinforce the effects of chemical sun protectors. Look out for antioxidants in any beauty product that you don't wash off – moisturisers, body lotions, sun creams and these days even make-up. If you live in a city, daily antioxidants are an absolute must – they will strengthen your skin's protection against the outside world.

OXYGEN We all know how glowing and radiant we look after a long, restorative walk in the countryside – so it was no surprise when oxygen started cropping up in face creams, too. As you'd expect, oxygen's job is to turbo-charge your skin's energy levels, making the cell renewal process work like clockwork and ensuring a fresh healthy layer of skin on the outside. However, oxygen is fairly unstable – there is no way of controlling when and how the oxygen molecules are released into the skin – and its effects might not last long after application. O2 facials are more effective – these usually take the form of an hour-long treatment involving the usual stages of deep-cleansing and skin-priming, before an oxygen fan is directed at your face for usually around twenty minutes. However, this is pretty expensive compared with a simple burst of outdoor exercise, which will have much the same effect.

LIPOSOMES These aren't ingredients so much as ingredient carriers. They've been around for a number of years now, but the technology required to construct them is so high-tech that they're mostly still available only in creams at the more expensive end of the market. They surround mole-cules of nutrients and other good things contained in the moisturiser and help them delve deeper into the skin than they would be able to on their own. They are particularly useful in anti-ageing products where more than surface-level moisturisation is needed.

COLLAGEN When collagen began appearing in moisturisers, you could almost hear the cheers in the beauty world. An extra dose of that naturally occurring wonder substance that gives our skin its firmness and elasticity? Yes please. But don't expect too much – it's impossible for a cream to deliver its collagen deep down where the skin needs it most. It should still have a noticeable effect on the surface, though, adding much-needed strength and vitality, particularly to ageing skins.

BOTANICALS There's nothing new about the use of botanicals or plant extracts in skincare – but it's important to remember that fresh discoveries are being made all the time (experts admit that only around a quarter of the world's plants have been studied, still fewer analysed for their benefits to the skin). Plant extracts are amazing as one ingredient often has multitudinous benefits for the skin – green tea is one of the biggest recent discoveries in skincare, and its abilities include free radical-fighting, skin renewing and radiance boosting.

MARINE As with plants, there are thousands of organisms in the ocean that are just waiting to be discovered. Seaweed is now a firm favourite among many skincare formulators, who were astounded by its ability to retain moisture and not dry out when washed up on a baking hot shore for long periods of time. Sea minerals are also big news – those that champion them hark back to evolutionary theory, saying we all began as aquatic creatures and that

the mineral content of sea water is very much in harmony with the mineral contents of our own bodies. Unsurprisingly then, marine products are particularly good for bathing and for the skin on our bodies, unless of course you're allergic to the iodine found in marine products.

ELEMENTS Sounds mad, but ingredients such as gold, silver and copper are big news in skincare. Not only do they have the obvious 'luxury' factor – which means the beauty companies are eager to use them – but they really can have a positive effect on your skin. The body already contains small quantities of some elements, such as copper, which helps the skin retain its strength. Silver has cleansing and anti-bacterial properties, while gold – unsurprisingly – is included for radiance boosting.

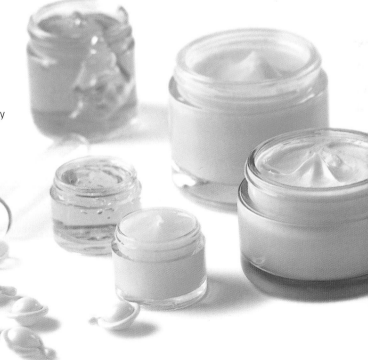

FUTURE PERFECT *So many beauty products, so little time! Familiarise yourself with the hi-tech jargon on labels – AHAs, liposomes, oxygen, etc. – to cut through the confusion and find out which is the best product for you and your lifestyle.*

between the lines

Do you see too many frown lines when you look in the mirror? In the fight against the dreaded wrinkles, a face-lift seems too drastic and creams take too long, so consider line fillers, cosmetic surgery's new middle ground. They're designed to 'melt away' age lines by using a variety of ultra-modern techniques that are quicker and less daunting than full facial surgery.

SMOOTH OPERATORS

As we age, skin starts to sag and wrinkle. Though traditional 'under-the-knife' surgery is still the only sure-fire way to eliminate sagging skin permanently (because the excess, 'baggy' skin is literally cut off), injections can now 'plump up' the skin so that the offending lines and creases are no longer clearly defined. The results aren't permanent – your body metabolises the injected substance within around three months – but they are immediate.

PLUMP UP YOUR SKIN

The most famous of the fillers are collagen injections. Collagen occurs naturally in the skin, and is responsible for keeping it firm and supple. Ageing and other factors, such as smoking and excessive sun exposure, deplete the skin's natural collagen supplies, so adding a bit with injections can minimise wrinkles and return a look of 'youthfulness' to ageing skin. They're among the longest-lasting fillers – you should be able to see the effects for around three months – and they're particularly effective for nasolabial lines (running from the corner of the nose to the corner of the mouth). One word of warning, though – some people can have an allergic reaction to injected collagen, which comes from cows, so it's essential to have a test prior to your treatment.

For a longer-lasting effect, autologous fat injections are sometimes recommended (the process is sometimes called a microlipoinjection). Here, fat is taken from elsewhere on the body – usually the buttocks or thighs – and used as a 'filler' for the face. It's particularly effective for wrinkles, for dark, crêpey skin round the eyes and – since it's essentially boosting fat content – hollow cheeks. Using your own fat eliminates the risk of allergic reactions, but it does involve separate appointments for removing fat and then re-injecting it into the face, which can increase the risk of infection. Fat injections can also be permanent, but this procedure is more expensive, takes longer to perform and longer for the results to appear (swelling takes one to three weeks to go down).

Newer collagen alternatives do a similar job but claim to have less risk from allergic reactions, and can also be used for plumping up the lips. Some, such as Hylaform, are animal derivatives, so an allergy test is still required. Others, such as New-Fill® and Restylane® are synthetic. One note here about silicone injections, which are sometimes offered by surgeons, although they're not cleared for cosmetic use. Avoid them. It's difficult to tell whether your body will accept or reject the silicone, and there are also risks of the silicone travelling to other parts of the body, causing infection.

It's also possible to get permanent fillers. Their major advantage is not having to keep getting your face 'topped up' – but as they represent some of the newest developments in the 'filler' arena, they're not without their glitches. Most, such as Artecoll® and Evolution, are tiny synthetic beads suspended in a gel that, once injected, support the efforts of the skin's own hyaluronic acid, collagen and elastin, giving a feeling of naturally firm, healthy and younger-looking skin. SoftForm is slightly different – it's like a tiny drinking straw that is placed behind deep lines so that the ageing tissue can mingle with it. With any of these, there is a risk from the implants going hard or becoming infected – in which case they would have to be removed, a tricky process that could lead to a scar.

BOTOX® – RELAX YOUR WRINKLES

What fillers are to age lines, Botox® is to expression lines – such as those that are formed from habitual frowning or smiling. They're caused by the muscles beneath the skin's surface, so to eliminate them, surgeons paralyse the offending muscle so that it can no longer move. Botox® is a trade name for botulinum toxin, which is produced by the clostridium botulinum bacterium used to treat muscle spasms. As an anti-ageing treatment, it works best on the horizontal lines across the forehead, the vertical lines at the top of the nose and the nose-to-mouth lines. It does not work on wrinkles caused by deterioration of collagen and fibrin. Botox® wears off over time, so treatments have to be repeated, though they should not be done more frequently than every three months.

It's also worth noting that some women have experienced unpleasant side effects from Botox®. If the injection goes askew, the wrong muscle can sometimes be paralysed and you can end up with a twitch, squint or drooping eye. This wears off eventually – but can be quite traumatic in the meantime. When used to treat lines on the forehead, some women also dislike the fact that Botox® can leave them somewhat expressionless – literally unable to convey emotion on their faces. Many health professionals who are unfamiliar with the facial anatomy are now injecting Botox®, so make sure you find a properly trained and qualified practitioner.

Fillers at a glance

THE AMOUNTS you'll be quoted are often per syringe full of filler and, depending on your wrinkles, you may need two or three syringes-full. Make sure you check this out before you start.

Problem	Treatment	Lasts for...
Wrinkles/ nasolabial folds	Collagen injections	3 months
Crêpey skin/ hollow cheeks	Autologous fat injections	permanent
Frown lines	Evolution Botox®	3–6 months
Thin lips	Synthetic injection (e.g. Restylane)	3 months
Sagging skin	Permanent filler (e.g. Artecoll)	permanent

SURFACE ISSUES

Skin resurfacing essentially means removing the outer layer of skin, so that a fresh new layer can form (this takes around one month). How permanent the results will be depends on the depth of the problem. Minor wrinkles and pigmentation are generally only on the surface, so they can be eliminated completely, but scars and older wrinkles usually come from deeper down. They can be made less noticeable, but not banished entirely.

A SECOND SKIN?

If your skin is generally lacklustre, with a tired complexion, patchy and uneven skin tone, wrinkles and basic lack of radiance, your best option could be to go for the gentlest of the treatments: microdermabrasion, which is a bit like having your face sandblasted (gently, of course!). Tiny aluminium oxide particles are sent down a tube to gently lift away dead skin cells and stimulate new growth, but there are no long-term effects – it will last only around ten days. It's the younger, more timid sister of dermabrasion, where a surgical instrument (either a high-speed rotating brush or a diamond-coated wheel) removes upper layers of the skin to rid it of surface irregularities such as dark spots caused by sun damage, acne scars and even superficial wrinkles. This is much harsher, and unlike the 'micro' version can leave your skin red and oozing afterwards.

Another option is the chemical peel, a more extreme version of a 'fruit acid' facial. These peels, which are done in a doctor's office, literally remove the surface layer of the skin. None is a permanent solution, but all can, to a lesser or greater degree, improve the appearance of wrinkled, sun-damaged, blemished or unevenly pigmented skin. The mildest uses an AHA solution, though a stronger one than is found in over-the-counter cosmetic products. It stings a bit and more than one treatment may be required. The next step in intensity is the trichloroacetic acid peel, and the strongest uses phenol. These two can be very uncomfortable, both during and after the treatment. The skin is very sun-sensitive after these treatments, so sun should be avoided entirely for a while and then a sunblock is essential whenever you're outdoors. The milder the substance used, the quicker the recovery, but continued peeling, redness and swelling may persist for as long as two weeks.

Next comes laser resurfacing. A light beam vaporises the upper strata of the skin, with the surgeon able to control the level of light so that the precise depth can be reached. Lasers are so specific, and there are so many different types, that they can have many different uses. Normally, the choice is between a carbon dioxide laser for deeper wrinkles (this may also cause permanent lightening of the treated area) or an erbium laser for fine to moderate wrinkles and facial scarring. In the past, a patient's sun damage or pigmentation would have to be fairly severe for a surgeon to recommend this over one of the other methods, but new and gentler treatments have recently been developed. One, called FotoFacial, uses pulsed light, but it is not, strictly speaking, a laser. Cool Touch and N-Lite lasers do not penetrate as deeply as the carbon dioxide and erbium lasers, so they are better suited to crow's feet and superficial wrinkles, but they have a shorter recovery period. Whatever the method, all facial laser surgery involves a certain amount of skin sensitivity afterwards.

Laser skin resurfacing

SKIN RESURFACING can treat wrinkles, scars, uneven skin/pigmentation and spider veins.

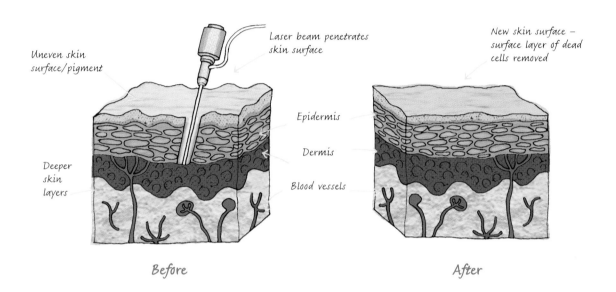

Laser beam penetrates skin surface

Uneven skin surface/pigment

New skin surface – surface layer of dead cells removed

Epidermis

Dermis

Blood vessels

Deeper skin layers

Before

After

MOLES, SCARS, BIRTHMARKS, SPIDER VEINS

Warts and skin tags are sometimes treated with lasers, but most effective for these is cryotherapy, where they are frozen off with the cold from liquid nitrogen. It's for scars, birthmarks and spider veins that lasers really come into their own (another surgical option for spider veins is sclerotherapy – *see pages 156–57*). There are no incisions, which means no scarring, and because lasers can be so accurately targeted, the risk of damage to the surrounding tissue is also minimal. The pain is like a hot needle, but if a large area is to be treated, your surgeon will recommend a light anaesthetic. With all laser treatments, it is important not to have a tan because the light from the laser beam is attracted to the melanin and it could cause damage to skin tissue. Most surgeons recommend waiting at least six weeks either before or after a holiday for an operation. It's usual to have a course of laser treatments, around four to eight weeks apart, until the treatment has been successful. Sometimes, treatment will plateau before the mark has completely disappeared and at this point your surgeon will end the course. For spider veins, the laser is used to seal off the burst blood vessels, which can usually be done in just one or two treatments. Superficial scars need similarly few treatments because they are located fairly close to the surface, but darker or deeper marks, such as port-wine stains and moles, may require up to eight treatments.

all mouth: help your teeth
Learning the tricks that lead to healthy teeth doesn't sentence you to a lifetime of sugar-free foods. It's all a question of knowing what, when and how to eat – and you'll soon realise that it is still possible to indulge your sweet tooth occasionally while still having teeth that are healthy and strong.

HEALTHY TEETH, HEALTHY BODY

Because they help us process food, it stands to reason that the food we eat has a direct bearing on the health (and appearance) of our teeth. But aesthetic issues aside, why is it so important that your teeth stay in good condition? Simple. There's a huge link between your oral health and overall health, with dental problems having strong links with medical conditions such as stroke, heart disease and diabetes.

DENTAL HYGIENE

Basically, a good dental hygiene routine is all about protecting against tooth decay and promoting periodontal health. Get that sorted, and the associated problems such as discolouration and sensitivity should (hopefully) take care of themselves. Of course, there are genetic issues surrounding things like the colour of your teeth, but at least this way you'll be giving yourself a flying start.

The good news is that, unlike other health regimes such as losing weight or building up fitness, even the most strict dental practice leaves a little room for treating yourself to some chocolate or a glass of cola every so often. We know that avoiding sugar is the first line of defence against tooth decay, but research shows that it's not actually so big a deal how much sugar you have in one sitting, but rather how frequently you eat it, and how long it stays in your mouth and, especially, in contact with your teeth.

'Basically, a good dental hygiene routine is all about protecting against tooth decay – and at the most fundamental level, that means thinking about what you eat.'

John F. Groombridge, Bachelor of Dental Surgery

Sugar in the mouth is metabolised by bacteria, which produces acid, lowering the pH values – this is when demineralisation happens (the dissolving of the tooth's enamel outer coating). A good rule of thumb is this: eat sugary foods or drinks only at mealtimes, when your mouth's pH levels are already being affected. Rinse your mouth with water after eating if you cannot brush your teeth until later. Avoid snacking on sweets between meals – but before you reach for the fruit bowl instead, remember that some fruits are worse for your teeth than sweets.

PREVENTATIVE MEASURES

Zesty citrus fruits such as oranges, lemons, limes and grapefruits are so acidic that they can actually cause tooth enamel to dissolve. Soft fruits are usually less of a worry, though experts are still not really sure why – it's thought to relate to whereabouts in the fruit's cells the sugar is stored. Another big no-no is fruit juice. Here, the sugars have been released from the cells and are at their most potent. If you love fruit juice, the best thing to do for your teeth (although perhaps not for your digestion) is to gulp it down — don't let it swish round your mouth for ages and definitely don't drink through a straw because it 'flushes' the liquid around your mouth.

How long you keep certain foods in your mouth is definitely an issue. As well as juices, it's also a good idea to keep an eye on sugary, sticky foods such as raisins, toffees, treacle and fruit gums, which adhere to your teeth in close proximity to plaque-forming bacteria, causing direct damage. Boiled sweets have a similarly prolonged attack. Also, don't think sugary carbohydrates are the only ones to avoid – although their acid content is lower, crisps and other savoury snacks are still poten-tially tooth-unfriendly.

A tooth-healthy food is one that provides calcium and phosphate to maintain the integrity of the tooth enamel, that has a low sugar content and that does not adhere to the teeth as many starchy foods (such as bread) do. The best thing to do is have fewer sessions of eating so the mouth is full of food less often during the course of a day, and to floss your teeth or at least

rinse your mouth with water after eating. If neither is possible, then chewing some sugar-free gum will stimulate the flow of saliva and rub food off the surface of the teeth. As a rule of thumb, try not to end your meals with a tooth-attacker. If you're having a sugary dessert, for example, be sure to follow it with some sugar-free gum. That way the offending ingredients won't get the opportunity to work on your teeth.

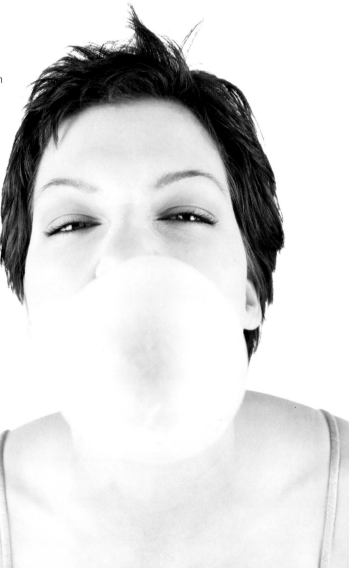

CHEW IT OVER *Chewing gum after meals will help neutralise the tooth-attack-ing acids in the mouth – but it has to be sugar-free!*

work that smile

Want a relaxed and natural grin? Make sure that your jaw's up to it by getting to know the warning signs that could mean jaw pain is on the way – neglecting the warning signals could lead to further health problems. Plus, if you're prone to jaw pain or tension, learn the exercise that will help your jaw to become firm and strong.

THROUGH CLENCHED TEETH...

If anyone's told you to grit your teeth and get on with it, they might not have your best interests at heart – especially not where your teeth and jaw are concerned. Clenching or grinding your teeth together – known as bruxism – puts pressure on the complex temporo-mandibular joint (or TMJ) and can lead to an array of symptoms that all come under the heading 'dental occlusion' (the word for teeth that do not meet correctly when your jaws bite together).

Chief among these symptoms is, unsurprisingly, jaw ache. Headaches, facial pain and even earaches are also common. The muscles get tired, and may even start going into spasm, which can not only be painful in itself but can also have a knock-on effect, causing pain in other parts of the body such as the back, neck and shoulders. Even yawning can be painful.

But if clenching your teeth is so bad, surely the best advice is simply to stop doing it? Unfortunately, it's not as simple as that. Studies show that the majority of people who clench or grind their teeth do so during sleep, so they don't even know that they're doing it. Times of extreme concentration and stress are also common for teeth clenching, and again this is a time when your mind is occupied elsewhere, making you less aware of your physical actions. Bruxism can also be caused by sleep problems and crooked teeth. So how is it possible to tell if you're a secret clencher or grinder? The biggest give-away is teeth sensitivity – especially when you've just woken up. If your early morning cup of coffee or ice-cold orange juice is creating a tingling sensation on your teeth, you could be experiencing the beginnings of dental occlusion problems. Further down the line, loose and broken fillings, teeth and crowns are common, as is generalised toothache with no apparent cause. Experiencing headaches first thing in the morning could also be another early wake-up call for teeth grinders, as could more generalised pain behind the eyes and in the neck and shoulders.

JAW RESCUE

The jaw itself is good at letting you know it's unhappy. The TMJ can become noisy, clicking and grating, and sluggish – reluctant to bite together for fear of pain. If you're concerned about any of these problems, consult your dentist – and try a few preventative measures at home.

Firstly, cut down your caffeine intake, which can tense muscles, and of course, stop chewing gum, which can put unnecessary pressure on your jaw. Secondly, actively try and relax your jaw muscles. Before you go to bed at night, hold two warm flannels to your jaw for several minutes, or until it feels relaxed. The idea is that this will make the jaw less tense and much more reluctant to work hard at clenching during the night.

In persistent cases of teeth grinding, your dentist can also fit a customised plastic night guard to protect your teeth. If this does not relieve your symptoms (which may take only a few weeks, but may take months) you might have to consider surgery. There are various options that are available: ultrasound and electrical stimulation send impulses into the jaw muscles to relax them, and repositioning or replacement operations for teeth are also effective options. Interestingly, Hormone Replacement Therapy has also been shown to ease dental occlusions in some women.

Finally, tailor your diet to the problem. While it is painful, make things easy for your jaw with soft foods – bananas instead of apples, yogurt instead of muesli. Switch back slowly as you try and refortify.

Jaw exercises

JAW EXERCISES are a good way to relieve jaw tension – or even as a preventative measure if you have no symptoms. Not only do they work the muscles, but done properly, they should also improve your head and neck posture, encouraging better muscle placement. If they feel painful, however, don't attempt them – your jaw clearly needs to rest, so you should skip this stage and go straight to your dentist.

1. Warm-up
Slowly open your jaw as wide as you can, and then close.
REPEAT up to ten times.

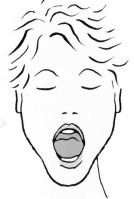

2. Mobility enhancer
Bite your teeth together. Open your jaw to only about 2.5 cm (1 inch). Without opening it any further, move it all the way to one side, then back to the centre.
REPEAT up to ten times and then swap sides.

3. Weight bearing
With two fingers pushing down on your lower teeth, slowly open your mouth as wide as you can.
REPEAT up to ten times.

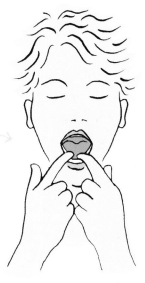

4. Stress reliever
Stand up straight with your arms by your side, shoulders soft and relaxed. Roll your head forward, keeping your spine straight and your abdominal muscles tucked in, then gently roll it up to one side, then back to the centre.
REPEAT, swapping sides.
REPEAT the whole sequence five times.

a brush with success
Maintaining clean, confidence-building teeth is like riding a bicycle – once you've cracked the routine, you never forget how. But is it that simple? Although most of us dutifully brush our teeth twice a day, it's amazing how easy it is to fall into bad habits.

THE BRUSH OFF *Brush twice a day for tip-top teeth. And less is more when it comes to toothpaste – a small blob is enough, because it's the brushing action that counts in the war against plaque.*

SPARKLING

You need to brush your teeth twice a day – upon awakening and before bed. There was a time when dentists recommended an even more diligent approach (after every mealtime) but now they feel that, in most cases, it's unrealistic and unnecessary to brush much more often – especially if you floss thoroughly every day as well.

When it comes to choosing the right toothpaste, as long as it contains fluoride, the difference between the vast array of gels and creams on offer is largely a matter of personal choice. Also, don't be fooled into thinking that more is better. You don't need to coat the length of the bristles – a small blob in the middle will be enough. It's the action of brushing your teeth, not the paste itself, that removes the plaque. Electric toothbrushes are also good if you have a tendency to rush when you brush – many have a timer (two to three minutes is about right). Sonic or powered toothbrushes that use sound waves are even better – but still quite expensive (around three times the price of a regular electric toothbrush). However, they may not be suitable for everyone – if you've got sensitive teeth, you could be better off with a regular toothbrush with soft bristles. For most people, toothbrushes labelled 'soft' or 'medium' are best.

SQUEAKY CLEAN

For maximum cleaning power, experts recommend holding the brush at 45 degrees to your gum line, and brushing gently with small circular movements over two or three teeth at a time – on the outside (the part of the crown you can see) and the inner tooth surface (hold your brush vertically to do this).

When it comes to mouth health, plaque is public enemy number one. This gummy paste of food, bacteria and mucus (yuck!) sticks to the surfaces and hides between your teeth, where it does enormous mischief. The bacteria eats into the enamel, causing tooth decay, and irritates and may even infect the gums. Combined with the old food, this bacterial action produces bad breath. Clearly, getting rid of plaque, on a daily basis, should be at the top of your list. The best way to do that is a combination of regular, thorough brushing and effective flossing.

Flossing can be a big bore, and it will make your gums bleed the first few times you do it. All the same, it's a must. To floss quickly and effectively, gently slide the floss between two teeth until you hit gum at the top. Don't concentrate the pressure of the floss on the gum – the moment when you feel the gum is when you should transfer the pressure to the sides of the teeth, moving the floss side to side as you work down the tooth, away from the gum. Ask your dentist or dental hygienist to instruct you in proper flossing techniques.

'Flossing daily or even twice daily is advisable. Plaque doesn't only affect teeth – it can also irritate gums, leaving them sore and tender.'
John F. Groombridge, Bachelor of Dental Surgery

There are a plethora of flosses available – if you have crowns or bridges, it's worth investing in a special tougher floss especially for these, as they need especially thorough cleaning to prevent infection and gum disease. Flosses that claim to glide easily between teeth are good, but the slippery surface can sometimes make them difficult to grab onto.

SWEET-SMELLING

Ending your brushing session with a few quick sweeps with your toothbrush over your tongue will feel strange at first – but this can remove unwanted bacteria and freshen breath. For the really committed, there are also tongue scrapers, which sound like medieval torture instruments but are actually painless – usually a plastic handle with a curved edge that does the scraping. The tongue's rough surface means bacteria can get trapped there, decaying and causing odour (it's estimated that up to 80 per cent of bad breath emanates from the tongue). Scraping your tongue removes the decaying plaque. Work back to front, scraping a few times each morning for optimum results.

Mouthwash can also give you that extra burst of fresh-breath confidence. The anti-bacterial properties of mouthwashes mean they can penetrate deeper layers of plaque that can't be accessed by brushing, and they can also wash away any bacteria that has been dislodged by brushing. However, choose a mouthwash carefully. 'Antiseptic' washes are often formulated with a large amount of alcohol, which is potentially drying for the mouth and, after short-term odour fighting, can make the problem of mouth odour worse. Those containing chlorine dioxide, sodium chlorite or zinc are thought to be more effective all-day solutions.

whiter than white

If you don't have perfectly white teeth – and let's face it, who does? – you can eliminate discolouration and flash a winning smile with the best new whitening techniques. From hardworking toothpastes to high-tech lasers, the modern methods to bleach your teeth promise a movie-star white smile without causing any sensitivity. Prepare to dazzle.

HOW BRIGHT IS YOUR SMILE?

If your teeth are more beige than gleaming white, don't worry – you're not alone. It's just that for some people, having less-than-pristine pearlies can become such a problem that they avoid showing their teeth as much as they can – which means no smiling, and this in turn means they don't look – or feel – as relaxed and confident as they could.

CAUSES OF DISCOLOURATION

Unhelpfully, there's no one single cause of tooth discolouration. Genetics play a part in how long your teeth maintain their original bright, white colour. Some people are simply born with a more off-white enamel – medications such as tetracycline preparations, for example, can cause tooth discolouration in the newborn's teeth when given to pregnant women. Excess fluoride intake during childhood can cause a yellow to brown staining known as fluorosis. Some diseases can also affect the way the body uses calcium, which can lead to white spots on the teeth.

Having said all that, there are of course other factors that can contribute to teeth discolouration – ageing, shock and nerve degeneration are some of the least controllable. Dietary perils such as coffee, cola and red wine, and tobacco use should all be kept to a minimum if you're trying to preserve teeth whiteness. It goes without saying that those stains you've created yourself are easier to remove than those that are genetic, but you can now make serious improvements even with more permanent discolouration.

QUICK-FIX SOLUTIONS

There are three levels of tooth whitening available: power whitening, which your dentist will carry out; at-home whitening procedures, which your dentist may give you or you can buy at the chemist; and whitening toothpastes. Power whitening lightens both the enamel and dentine in the tooth, so it is the most effective. It uses a strong bleaching agent, so your gums must be protected by a special shield. First, an oxygen-releasing whitening gel is painted over the surfaces of the teeth. Next, an intense light is directed at the whitening gel to activate the oxygenating process. The oxygen whitens the coloured substances, and only the colour is made whiter, while the structure of the teeth is unchanged. The whole procedure should take no more than an hour, but you may be required to wear a custom-made tray filled with the oxygen gel at night for the following couple of weeks.

However, smoking and eating those 'danger' foods again will take the edge off your new bright, white teeth (dentists will advise eating only non-pigmented foods, such as bread, pasta, mashed potato and yogurt, for the first twenty-four hours after treatment), and there is also evidence to suggest that this kind of bleaching process can make your teeth slightly more susceptible to staining in the future. In any case, most teeth-whitening procedures benefit from a follow-up treatment every year or so, although this often simply involves wearing the oxygen-gel mouth guard.

It's also worth noting that fillings, crowns and veneers are immune to the effects of whitening procedures (although veneers in particular are difficult to stain). After the treatment, they may end up looking darker than your shiny new teeth and you might want to consider having them replaced to get a truly uniform look. For spot-stains, micro-abrasion is sometimes used – the stained areas are literally sanded off – although this technique is really only effective for very superficial stains.

At-home bleaching kits are popular, but the results can be variable. They sometimes enhance, rather than mask variations in enamel colour and can also increase tooth sensitivity. They use a bleaching gel and a mouth tray to keep the bleach in contact with your teeth. The bleach used in most whitening techniques is typically peroxide, which is also mildly irritating to the soft tissues in the mouth. At-home kits are usually not potent enough to be harmful, but if you do experience stinging, rinse immediately with salt water. The most lifestyle-friendly are those you wear overnight for around a fortnight, but you can get twice-daily varieties, too.

Finally, whitening toothpastes. They contain mild abrasives that literally clean and polish, with added chemical agents to turbo-charge the stain-removal process. They will not, though, change the colour of your teeth.

Whiter teeth – the cheat's guide

MAKE-UP can do wonders to enhance your teeth's natural colour. A fake tan or bronzer will give you a healthy glow and provide a good contrast between your skin colour and your teeth. If you want to play down your mouth, play up your eyes. As the two 'wet' areas of the face, they are the most prominent, so bring your eyes to the fore with a shimmering eyeshadow and lashings of mascara.

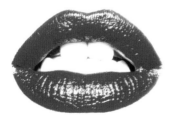

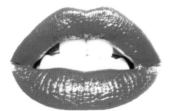

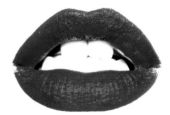

Choose cool-toned lipsticks, such as bright reds and blue-based pinks, to make teeth stand out.

Steer clear of brown and peachy tones, which can make your teeth look more yellow.

Go for matt rather than gloss formulations, which will draw attention towards the lip area.

TEETH FOR LIFE

Think of major dental work and most of us run screaming – but arming yourself with the facts is the first step towards learning that dental surgery need be no more scary than any other kind. The second step is finding a dentist you trust. He or she must be registered with the General Dental Council and, although not mandatory, most dentists are members of the British Dental Association. You should be able to have a consultation to discuss your concerns without paying. You should also be able to take away leaflets to study without feeling pressurised to make an appointment there and then. Depending on the work you're having done, it's worth asking if your dentist has a specialism in that area, or at the very least performs the procedure on a regular basis. Ask for specific prices first – many operations have follow-up procedures, which could become expensive.

A GUIDE TO DENTAL PROCEDURES

DENTAL AMALGAMS The most common procedure you're likely to encounter is the plain old filling – or to give it its more impressive title, dental amalgam. The oldest and most familiar variety is a silver-coloured amalgam that contains mercury. These have been the focus of debate recently, with some people suggesting that the mercury could migrate elsewhere in the body. As a result, mercury fillings are now banned in Switzerland and some US states. There have been some cases of allergies from mercury fillings, although the American Dental Association insists that only around 100 cases of allergy have ever been reported.

If you're at all worried about the silver mercury amalgams, however, there are other options available. Tooth-coloured fillings are a composite of glass and resin, and have the added advantage of blending in well with the

Dental veneers and implants

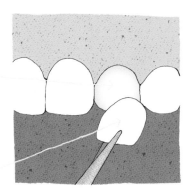

Existing tooth – discoloured or chipped

Veneer (made of porcelain or plastic) is adhered to damaged tooth

Veneer

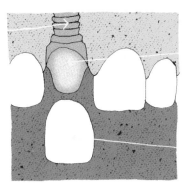

Broken tooth is removed and metal screw-like implant is fitted – this fuses with the jawbone

Abutment – an extension to the implant

New crown is attached to the abutment

Implant and crown

DISCOLOURED or chipped teeth can be disguised with veneers; badly broken or missing teeth can be replaced with an implant and crown.

rest of your teeth. Many people opt for these when fillings are needed at the front of the mouth, but settle for the amalgam type at the back – composite resins are more expensive (usually around three times the price of mercury fillings, and not thought to be as strong). The same resin substance can also be used for restoring slightly chipped or worn teeth – this is known as bonding.

'Experiments with laser technology mean that in the future, it's possible that amalgams will be a lot less common than they are now.'
John F. Groombridge, Bachelor of Dental Surgery

Some dentists are predicting that tooth decay and fillings will one day be a lot less common than they are currently. New experiments with laser technology suggest that it may be possible to detect the beginnings of dental erosion before it's even had a chance to penetrate the enamel (outer layer). Any damage done would therefore be superficial and solved by thorough cleaning and spot-treating.

One downside of fillings is that they often need replacing after a while (usually ten years) – even if they're not causing any trouble. Daily activities such as chewing and clenching can cause wear and tear on fillings, plus food and bacteria can also sometimes tunnel their way beneath the filling, causing further damage to the tooth and meaning a larger filling than before is now required.

CROWNS AND IMPLANTS When a tooth is so decayed that there isn't enough left to support both itself and the filling, a crown is what's required. It's like a permanent façade for your tooth, and is a useful way of covering and protect-ing teeth that are weak, broken or even discoloured (although crowns will not change colour after tooth-whitening procedures). When one or more teeth are missing, a bridge can be made and attached to supporting teeth on either side of the gap. The bridge consists of one or more 'false teeth' with a metal piece that hooks around the back of the supporting teeth. Bridges can be permanent or removable. If the supporting teeth are not strong enough to hold the bridge, they may be covered with a crown.

Another option for a missing or extremely weak tooth is to replace it with an implant covered by an artificial tooth. Implants involve quite a lengthy surgical process and are not suited to everyone. A metal post is placed into the jawbone and left for up to six months while bone grows around it in order to anchor it firmly. Then an artificial tooth is fitted over the post.

VENEERS In order to transform the appearance of the teeth, veneers are also an option. They're more likely to be recommended for serious discolouration in certain individual teeth than for a more generalised colour problem, but can also be applied to every tooth. You'd be likely to go for veneers instead of tooth whitening if you wanted a longer-lasting effect – you'll usually get up to ten years' wear from them. They are thin shell-like covers that are permanently attached to the front of the tooth. There are two main types: resin veneers that can be applied in one sitting, or porcelain veneers that take two or three appointments. The porcelain ones are more expensive, but retain their colour better. Veneers change not only the colour of your teeth but also how they feel inside your mouth. They usually take a few weeks to get used to.

well-fed hair

Can what you eat really make a difference to your hair? Talk as much as you like about strong hair, healthy hair, soft hair or manageable hair – there's only one thing any of us really wants: shiny hair. And while there are dozens of shine-imparting gels and sprays available, we all know that the only way to get a shine that lasts for days, not hours, is by nourishing your hair from within.

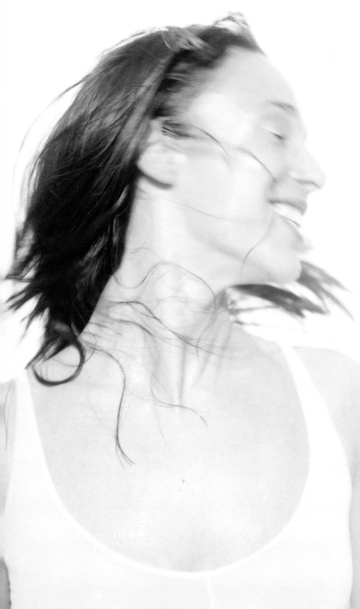

HAIR NUTRITION

Hair changes according to what feeds it. That includes the environment, the products you use, your levels of stress and fatigue and – perhaps above all – your diet. But before you dismiss the idea of embarking on a special reviving diet as at best optimistic and at worst unrealistic, don't worry. Eating your way to shinier hair couldn't be easier, and if you're trying to eat healthily anyway, you're probably already doing everything you should. The only caveat to eating well for your hair is that glossy hair takes time to achieve naturally – you may see an instant difference, but it could be a couple of months before you see the results you want every day. Unlike skin, hair cannot repair itself, so you have to wait for newer, healthier hair to grow through.

For general improvements, there are a few key nutritional points to note. The first – and golden – hair rule is to drink plenty of water. Without it, all the nutrients in the world aren't going to make it easily into your growth-inducing hair follicles. Because hair is around 90 per cent protein, the next big thing is to make sure you're eating enough protein (you need around 50 grams (2 oz) of protein daily for healthy hair, skin and nails). Iron is also essential to combat hair loss (a particular problem for vegetarians and those suffering from thrush) and with iron comes the need for vitamin C, which can boost your body's iron-processing abilities. Fresh, fresh, fresh fruit and vegetables should always be on the menu.

For more targeted problems, consider supplements. To combat dry, brittle hair, increase the protein in your diet and consider a supplement of cod liver oil. Ageing (greying) hair could be helped with a supplement of amino acids. To boost your hair's thickness and lustre, take essential fatty acids. For hair growth, stock up on energy-inducing B vitamins. If hair loss is the concern, increase your intake of fresh vegetables and consider taking extra vitamins A and H, but as with all supplements, excessive doses should be avoided.

HAIR FOR LIFE

Each hair follicle is entirely separate, growing and 'resting' independently of all the others in a process that takes up to five years, before the hair shaft is shed to make way for a new one. If too many of the follicles start working in sync, this will result in mass hair loss – which is exactly what can happen at certain times in our lives.

In the same way that your hair reflects the condition of your health, increasing evidence shows that it also mirrors your state of mind. Stress can be a major cause of hair loss. A condition called telogen effluvium causes large-scale hair loss that appears as thinning hair radiating outwards from the part and eventually involving the entire scalp. Stresses ranging from emotional upset to childbirth, crash dieting (especially with inadequate protein) to high fever can bring on telogen effluvium. What happens is this: at any given time, 90 per cent of the hairs on your head are in their growing phase (anagen) and 10 per cent have shut down (telogen) and are resting before being pushed out by a new hair growing beneath it. Stress forces as much as 30 per cent of the hair into telogen and you lose on average 300 hairs a day. It all adds up to very thin hair over the course of a few months. The good news is that the hair growth normalises once the stress has been removed or the underlying cause treated.

'Hair is one of the best barometers for your body's general health. How it looks can be seen as its reaction to the things that feed it: oxygen and nutrients from the blood supply, and good circulation. They can only get there if you eat them!'
Marilyn Sherlock, Chair of the Institute of Trichologists, London

Illness can be a cause of hair loss, too – particularly thyroid problems – but much of your hair's behaviour is also due to hormonal factors. The loss of appetite that often ensues with illness simply adds to the problem. Hair often looks healthier than ever during pregnancy, and opinion is somewhat divided as to why. Some experts say it's due to the surge of oestrogen in your body (oestrogen inhibits hair loss), which would explain why the birth control pill is sometimes reported to have a similar effect. Others attribute it to the fact that during pregnancy, most women are practising healthier eating habits – keeping alcohol to a minimum, for example. After giving birth, though, most women can expect to notice a dip in their hair's condition and even significant hair loss. At this point, it is important to make sure you're eating enough protein and fresh fruit and vegetables so that the new hair that grows through will be twice as lustrous.

exercising for good hair

Some workouts are great for your hair, some are not so good. Either way, you don't have to forego your fitness regime if you follow these simple guidelines. Hair thrives when it's lavished with lots of care and attention, so after exercise don't just wash and leave – give your hair the attention that it deserves. Read on for the best haircare tips.

HAIR WORKOUT

Let's get one thing straight: regular exercise is fantastic for your hair. Your hair thrives on a plentiful supply of blood, oxygen and nutrients, and the best way to deliver these is with the kind of turbo-charged circulation system that only an effective fitness regime can bring. It's just that some methods are better than others.

THE IMPACT OF EXERCISE

Yoga is the shining light of the hair-enhancing fitness regimes. Perfect the headstand (Shirshasana) and you'll be encouraging an unprecedented blood supply to your hair and scalp, resulting in shinier hair that even grows faster, too. If a headstand is too strenuous, you can try the cheat's method: just hang your head over the bath for a few moments when you wash it.

The gym is not somewhere traditionally associated with fabulous hair, but it can definitely have its uses. Some women apply a rich conditioner to the very tips of their hair before pinning it up for their workout, maximising its conditioning action with the body heat that their exercising will generate. However, you should avoid putting styling products on your scalp before a workout: in the same way that face creams can clog up a perspiring face, hair preparations will block the pores on your scalp, leading to oily hair and an irritated and flaky scalp.

For most of us, the effects of swimming on hair are all too familiar. Straw-like strands that look bleached out and dull are par for the course with most regular swimmers, and even wearing a hat doesn't provide total protection as water can often seep in through the edges. The problem with chlorine is two-fold: firstly, if it's left on the hair, it has a similar bleaching effect to peroxide (the substance used in professional hair-lightening products); secondly, like peroxide, chlorine can penetrate the outer layer of the hair (cuticle) and head straight for the inner shaft, where all the vital nutrients are housed.

To combat the drying and fading effects of chlorine, you need to find a shampoo that's also able to penetrate the cuticle. Specific swimming and many sun haircare products can do this, as well as many moisturising shampoos. Wash your hair immediately after swimming and, because these shampoos are so adept at penetrating hair, condition afterwards with a super-nourishing conditioner.

Once a week, treat hair to a hydrating 'mask' – you can buy special ones or use a rich conditioner and leave it on for five or ten minutes before rinsing. It will give hair a chance to top up its moisture levels properly for the week ahead.

HAIRCARE FOR LIFE

Take the lottery out of looking after your hair with these fail-safe ways to care for it.

WASH WELL It's no longer necessary to shampoo and rinse twice – traditional thinking was that you washed once to remove dirt, then once to cleanse and soften. Many modern shampoo formulations are clever enough to do both. Follow with a conditioner, but unless your hair is seriously parched, confine it to the mid-lengths and ends of your hair. Leave-in conditioners are also good, especially if you're in a hurry, but they're best for those with normal to dry hair.

DRY WELL Let your hair dry naturally as often as you can. Pat (not rub) with a towel first to remove excess water (ultra-absorbent towels are fantastic for this). When you blow-dry, use the lowest setting and start with the roots, working the nozzle down the hair shaft (to keep the fibres smooth). Hold the dryer at least 10 cm (4 inches) away from your hair.

BRUSH WELL Brush wet hair only if you really must – otherwise wait until it's half dry. When wet, use only a wide-toothed comb: your hair swells to twice its natural size when wet, and won't take kindly to being dragged through a fine-toothed one.

STYLE WELL Styling products that contain silicones are heat-protective, so use these before blow-drying. To style hair when dry, choose a textured product, such as gel, wax

or pomade (a kind of dry wax) on short or thick hair and serum or sprays on hair that's long or fine. Whatever consistency you're using (even sprays), get a natural look by rubbing the product all over the palms of your hands first. If you're worried you've taken too much, rub off the excess and apply to the underneath of your hair first, where it won't be so noticeable.

GLEAMING *Treat your hair in the same way as you would your skin – regular doses of TLC will ensure your locks are glossy and gorgeous.*

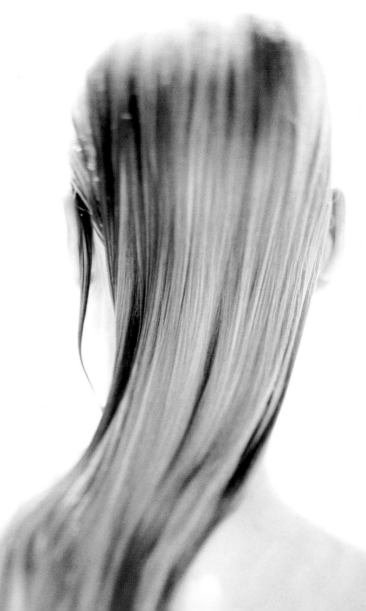

define your style

More than ever, it's not necessary to be content with the head of hair nature gave you. Thanks to modern techniques, it's possible to change your style as often as you like and experiment with different colours, too. Hair dyes were once the preserve of the prematurely grey, but nowadays formulations are so good that everyone can express themselves with colour.

STYLE

Whatever your hair's length, regular trims (every six to eight weeks) are the key to keeping it healthy. Snipping off the dry ends regularly prevents them from splitting and means that health-giving nutrients can penetrate right to the hair's tip. After that, it's regular washing and conditioning that will make all the difference. You can work out your hair type by running your fingers along a single strand of hair and feeling whether it's oily or dry and porous (it can be a combination of both – oily at the root, dry at the end is most common).

Most people find they need to detangle the older hair at the ends, where the cuticles don't lie flat, with conditioner. Ragged ends also have difficulty reflecting the light, resulting in a dull appearance. Conditioner comes to the rescue by coating them in a waxy layer that smoothes out these edges, promoting healthy, gleaming locks.

Whether your hair is naturally straight or curly is something you can't change (it's determined by the shape of your hair follicles), but these days it can be transformed in an instant. For curly hair, straightening irons can give sophisticated poker-straight styles that will last until your next wash, and for something more permanent, in-salon chemical straightening (which literally works exactly the opposite to a perm) can last for several months.

For natural-looking curls, there are several options. Perms have come on in leaps and bounds since the tight 'corkscrew' curls of the 1980s (gentle waves are now an option), but if your hair is colour-treated (dyed hair is already weak and it could start to break off) or if permanent curls are too drastic for you – don't perm. For one-night-only curls, try out curling tongs or hot brushes. Ironically, many hairdressers recommend blow-drying your hair straight before tonging so that you're starting with a totally clean 'canvas' to work on, and remember that the tighter you wind hair round, the smaller and tighter the curls. It's always advisable, though, to make them a little tighter than you really want in order to let hair 'drop' throughout the day.

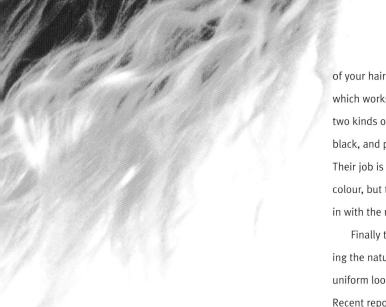

of your hair – they contain low levels of hydrogen peroxide, which works by altering hair's melanin levels. Hair contains two kinds of melanin – eumelanin, which is dark brown/black, and pheomelanin, which creates blonde or red tones. Their job is still basically to add shine and enhance natural colour, but they can also help to blend the first signs of grey in with the rest of the hair. They last for up to six weeks.

Finally there are permanent dyes. They work by changing the natural pigment found within the hair and give a uniform look to the hair (bleach lightens, dye darkens). Recent reports have linked sustained use of permanent hair dyes to bladder cancer because of ingredients known as arylamines. Darkest dyes are most potent as they contain the strongest chemicals, and using them as often as once a month could be cause for concern. Talk to your hairdresser about natural dark dyes such as henna.

Unless you're making a serious fashion statement, hair dyes should look natural. Initially, don't stray more than two or three shades lighter or darker than you were to begin with, or consider highlights or lowlights, where permanent dye is applied only to certain strands of hair. This works particularly well for giving dark blonde hair a 'sun-lightened' effect. Most people find they need to go and have their 'parting sprinkled' (roots redone) around every six weeks to hide that tell-tale regrowth.

One of the most popular looks is the 'naturally sun-lightened' look – it's a bit like fake tan for your hair. Have highlights done just one or two shades lighter than your usual colour, and restrict them to the top of your head and the sections of hair that frame your face – anywhere the sun would hit.

LOVE YOUR COLOUR

It's now estimated that 50 per cent of all women apply some sort of colour treatment to their hair, and today's colourants run the gamut from wash-in, wash-out treatments to there-till-it-grows-out dyes. As well as permanent treatments, salons are now starting to offer semi-permanent treatments too, describing them as 'shine boosters' or 'colour fresheners'. Sometimes these contain chemicals, but sometimes they're what's known as a 'vegetable rinse' – plant extracts that contain natural hair stains.

If you want to start with a softly, softly approach, you won't be able to drastically alter your hair colour, but you can enhance what nature gave you. Semi-permanent colours wash out within six to eight shampoos and act as a stain for the hair shaft – they don't penetrate the outer layer. They're good for creating a brighter (not lighter) look by bringing natural highlights to the fore, and work especially well on mid-brown tones. Demi-permanent colourants are the mildest of the dyes that actually alter the structure

WHEN HAIR MEETS SKIN

Stress is fast becoming one of the most widely recognised causes of hair problems. Of course, as well as the mental stress that we all know about, hair can be 'stressed' by many other factors, such as dirt, pollution, blow-drying, styling products and a poor diet.

FLAKY SCALP

Dandruff, particularly, is increasingly being associated with signs of mental stress: it's thought to inhibit the skin's ability to shed and renew itself, meaning that dead skin cells cling to the surface of the scalp, using up vital moisture supplies and leaving the fresh new layer underneath dry and parched. This causes the scalp to produce more oil to compensate for the dryness, and before you know it, that oil has mingled with the flaky old, dead cells, joining them together to create larger, greasy flakes. Most people think that dandruff is the result of a dry scalp and can't understand why their hair feels oily, but actually it's oil that's the cause. Anti-dandruff shampoos can be incredibly effective. Wash your hair in warm, not hot, water and you should also avoid applying silicone-based styling products to your scalp – they smother the skin, making the 'shedding' process even harder.

HAIR LOSS

As we get older, hair thins out – by the age of fifty, half of all women will have noticed some degree of hair thinning. Like male-pattern baldness (androgenic alopecia), hair loss in women is related to hormonal shifts, especially after menopause. Hair growth-promoting preparations containing minoxidil offer varying degrees of success, but they work only as long as you continue using them.

Hair transplants (or 'grafts') are now very common and are particularly good for rejuvenating small, patchy areas of hair growth. Under local anaesthetic, a surgeon will remove small patches of scalp from areas with good hair growth, and graft them on to hair-loss areas. The number of hairs that can be transplanted in one go varies enormously, but generally about fifty 'plugs' of hair are moved in one go. Plugs also differ in size, usually ten to fifteen hairs constitute one plug, but a mini-graft contains two to four hairs and a micro-graft, one to two hairs. Flap surgery is better for large, blanket areas of scalp – a section of scalp is cut out and replaced with a flap of hair-bearing skin (from elsewhere on the scalp) that remains connected to its original blood supply.

All hair-replacement techniques work with your existing hair, so it's important that you have a healthy supply on some parts of your head – normally the back or the sides. It's also important to remember that you'll never be able to recreate the amount of coverage you once had – it's more a question of damage limitation, covering the areas where most hair has been lost. This can sometimes leave a patchy effect.

With age, your whole hair-growth process slows down. Hair doesn't grow as fast, individual strands become finer, and the follicles produce less melanin, meaning they look lighter and give the illusion of being less in number. When your hair starts to grey is basically a matter of genetics, but most people begin noticing those silvery strands in their thirties. It's not possible to return hair to its original colour,

Hair growth cycle

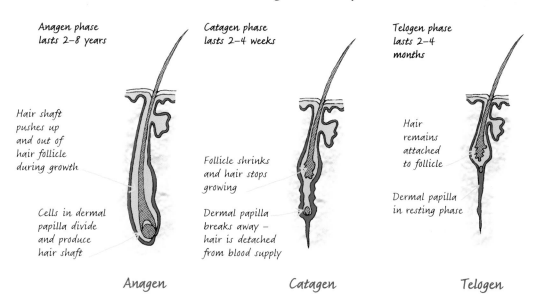

Anagen phase
lasts 2–8 years

Catagen phase
lasts 2–4 weeks

Telogen phase
lasts 2–4
months

Hair shaft
pushes up
and out of
hair follicle
during growth

Follicle shrinks
and hair stops
growing

Hair
remains
attached
to follicle

Cells in dermal
papilla divide
and produce
hair shaft

Dermal papilla
breaks away –
hair is detached
from blood supply

Dermal papilla
in resting phase

Anagen

Catagen

Telogen

GROWTH PHASES Normal hair growth goes through three phases: anagen (growing), catagen (transition) and telogen (resting). After the telogen phase, the cycle returns to the anagen phase and the new hair shaft pushes the old hair out.

which is why most people who are concerned about going grey opt for some form of dye treatment – either on selected sections or the whole head of hair.

HOLISTIC HAIR

Whether you've had scalp surgery or not, it's clear that for healthy hair, your scalp can benefit from as much TLC as you want to offer. The resurgence of interest in Ayurveda, an ancient Eastern belief system, has brought with it a renewed focus on the head and scalp – body parts that in Ayurveda play a vital role in healing and relieving pain. The philosophy is that by oxygenating the cells of the scalp, you will get the lymph system moving and release physical and emotional toxins, thereby calming the mind, clearing out the body and improving the appearance of your face and hair. It's one of the most relaxing treatments available, with deep finger pressure on the neck, scalp and face, and long, soothing strokes on the arms and back. For a self-scalp massage, wet hair, then place your fingertips crab-like above your ears and, without moving them, make rotating movements with them. Move your hands to your forehead, nape of your neck and finally temples. It needn't take long – just after you've rinsed out the shampoo when you're in the shower would be an ideal time. Afterwards, wrap your hair in a towel and relax for a few moments – particularly nice last thing at night.

eyes fit to look through

They're super-expressive, and one of our most noticeable features, yet do we really give our eyes the attention they deserve? Modern life – computer screens, pollution, stress and so on – can lead to tired, strained and irritated eyes, so spare a thought for them in your diet, lifestyle and even exercise routine.

DIET

When it comes to the vitamins and minerals that are good for your eyes, there's no doubt about it: antioxidant vitamin A (retinol and beta-carotene) is right at the top of the list. True, it's also fabulous for your hair and skin, but it's in the eyes that it really comes into its own – in developing countries, vitamin A deficiency is the biggest (preventable) cause of blindness. It prevents night blindness, ulceration of the cornea and dry eyes. With a regular supply of fresh fruit and vegetables, it's quite easy to get the RDA (Recommended Dietary Allowance) of vitamin A (600mcg) – you'll get your daily need from an average-sized carrot.

Mangoes, sweet potatoes, spinach and other colourful fruits and vegetables are great fresh sources, and liver, milk, eggs, butter and cheese have some, too.

Other antioxidants are also important – most eye complaints start because of free radical damage that antioxidants can help to combat. Vitamins C and E, plus the mineral selenium are excellent free radical–fighters (*see pages 30–31*). A plentiful supply of water is essential because it lubricates the eye, preventing dryness and discomfort. While we're talking about other good measures for general health, it would be good to give cigarette smoke a wide berth, too – it more than doubles your risk of cataracts.

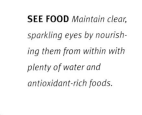

SEE FOOD *Maintain clear, sparkling eyes by nourishing them from within with plenty of water and antioxidant-rich foods.*

EXERCISE

If eating the right foods for your eyes is preventative, then eye exercises can certainly be curative. Not only can they relieve the kind of imperceptible eye strain that's caused by computers, televisions and harsh strip lighting, they can also aid some of the associated symptoms, such as head and neck aches. Still need convincing? For those concerned with wrinkles, eyestrain is also thought to be a major contributor to crow's feet.

If you work at a computer, taking mini 'eye breaks' every ten minutes or so is a must to prevent strain – look away from the screen at something 4–6 m (15–20 feet) away. Going one better, by leaving your desk and spending a few moments outside, will also do your eyes the world of good. It will return your eyes to natural light, meaning they don't need to work as hard, and will also give them a break from moisture-sapping air-conditioning. Ever wondered why you yawn so much at work? Experts believe it's partly to do with the fact that it pro-duces tears that help lubricate dry eyes. And you thought you were just bored. Also, drink lots of water throughout the day – if you're well hydrated, eyes will be adequately lubricated and they won't feel so dry and tired.

One of the best eye exercises to rejuvenate tired eyes and give those intraocular eye muscles an aerobic workout is to spend a minute or so looking up and then down, and then another minute looking from left to right. Sometimes it helps to focus on a particular spot at each side – that way it's easier to establish a regular pattern. More advanced than this is the 'focusing' exercise. Hold one of your fingers (or a pencil) about 2.5 cm (1 inch) away from your face, then slowly move it further and further away until your arm is outstretched. Now look beyond your finger into the dis-tance. Slowly reverse the process until your finger is back near your face. Repeat it several times. If you're worried about eyestrain, try to do both of these once a day, blinking several times in between to relax the muscles.

Palming exercise

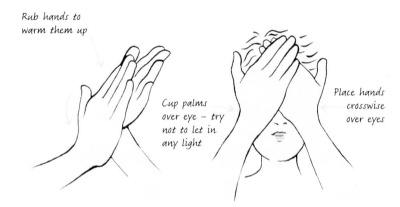

Rub hands to warm them up

Cup palms over eye – try not to let in any light

Place hands crosswise over eyes

Palming EYE REJUVENATING

If you've been working on screen all day, this is a quick and easy exercise that you can do at your desk. Rub your hands together to warm them up. Once they're warm, cup them over your eyes with your fingers crossed over your fore-head. Leave for five or ten minutes.

In yoga, 'palming' means rubbing your palms until they're warm and then cupping them over your eyes, with your fingers crossing over on your forehead (*see above*). Be careful not to bend your head forward – sitting on the floor with your elbows resting on your drawn-up knees encourages good posture for this.

Mirrors can also help you exercise your eyes. Focus on an object in the mirror, then step backwards slowly, so the object appears to be moving further away. Retreat a good few paces, then walk forward and keep focusing on the object as it gets nearer. Finally, when you're out and about, look all around you – above, below and right into the dis-tance – you'll be amazed how much more you notice. And at home, make sure you're never closer than 1.8 m (6 feet) to the TV – especially if you've been sitting at a computer all day.

EYES FIT TO LOOK AT

As our most expressive feature, it's only natural that we should want our eyes to look stunning at all times. Before you even think about your eyes themselves, take a look at your brows – sometimes even a simple reshape can 'lift' your face so much you could trick friends into thinking you've had surgery. Simple expert shaping tips are these: Pluck from beneath your brow line, never at the top. Draw an imaginary line upwards from the outer edge of your nostrils – your brows shouldn't extend much further in than this. If you're worried about shaping your brows yourself, book an appointment at a beauty salon. Once you've had your brows shaped once, you can follow the outline yourself at home. One brow treatment currently taking the beauty world by storm is threading – an ancient Indian art where the brows are pulled out with cotton. The advantage is that the hairs are pulled out at the root, meaning it's much longer before they grow back – up to two weeks.

LENSES AND GLASSES

If you wear glasses or contact lenses, you can also dramatically alter your appearance. With glasses, you should contrast your face shape with your frame shape. Round faces look best with oval frames, square faces with rounded ones and heart-shaped faces with narrow frames. Contact lenses now come in an array of colours and patterns – from pale tints that aid insertion (because you can see them better) to opaque lenses for dark eyes. You can even get non-prescription ones so that you can still experiment with eye colours even if you've got perfect sight. Light-filtering tints are fantastic for sports enthusiasts – they mute some

of the light spectrum so that certain colours (for example, yellow, for tennis balls) stand out. UV-blocking lenses are also available. These are no substitute for sunglasses (they protect only the cornea, not the whole eye, and eyelids in particular are at risk from burning), but the advantage is that the UV-blockers used are clear, meaning they won't affect your vision at all. One disadvantage of coloured lenses is that the coloured disc often slightly covers the iris, meaning vision could be impaired, so some eye experts prefer to limit them to non-regular use. As a rough guide, choose green, hazel or chestnut lenses if you have warm (peach-toned) colouring, and blue, grey or violet if your complexion is cooler (more pink).

A RAY OF LIGHT FOR VISION PROBLEMS

If your vision problems are caused by an irregularly shaped cornea (the clear covering over the front of the eye), then laser eye surgery could be for you. It's had a fair amount of bad press over the past few decades, but many of those painful, unpredictable and expensive original techniques have now been overtaken by a newer procedure called LASIK (Laser-Assisted In-Situ Keratomileusis). In this operation, a surgeon cuts a microfine flap from the clear covering of the eyeball, uses a laser to reshape the cornea so that it bends light rays precisely towards the retina again (a process called photoablation), then replaces the flap of tissue. The biggest advantages are that it is quick – the operation takes only about ten minutes per eye and the effects will become apparent in around twenty-four hours. And it is also relatively painless – most sensitivity lasts only for the first day or so after the operation.

As well as being quick, easy and painless, the good thing about LASIK eye surgery is that it can treat myopia (near-sightedness), hyperopia (farsightedness) and astigmatism (distorted vision) alike. With all three vision problems, the surgery works best when the loss of vision is fairly moderate. Vision can then be restored to at least 20/40. Some patients are also suitable for an 'enhancement' three months later, which can then achieve 20/20 (optimum) vision. The operation is less successful for people with either very weak or very strong prescriptions, and is also unsuitable for presbyopia, the age-related vision change that is due to a loss of flexibility of the lens. Other unsuitable candidates – and there are about one in ten – are those who are pregnant, those who have had previous eye injuries, or those who suffer from a serious health condition.

There are those who oppose LASIK treatment because they consider problems such as short-sightedness as conditions, not diseases or illnesses – akin to being taller or shorter than you'd like. They argue that the eye is too complex and valuable an organ to interfere with needlessly. But for some people, for whom glasses are diminishing their eyesight by encouraging dependence on them, or for those who simply don't like glasses and find contact lenses do not suit their lifestyle, LASIK surgery is a valuable option.

The biggest downsides to the surgery are the risks of infection and the problem of over-correction. Each patient will heal differently, which could alter the shape of the cornea – and that's something the surgeon can't predict. If you're considering eye treatment, it's vital to know the risks and talk to your surgeon so you can go into the operation with your eyes wide open.

LASIK eye surgery – how it works

LASIK (Laser-Assisted In-Situ Keratomileusis) can be used to treat nearsightedness, farsightedness and astigmatism – although this type of surgery isn't suitable for severe cases. The procedure is simple and takes only around ten minutes.

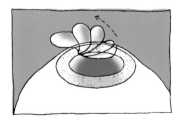 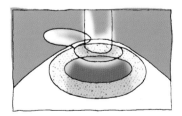 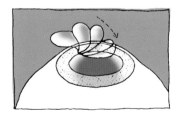

1. The patient receives a few drops of anaesthetic in the eye. Then an extremely fine flap of corneal tissue is cut and lifted away from the eye.

2. The laser is directed onto the cornea and remodels its shape to treat nearsightedness, farsightedness or astigmatism. This procedure lasts only 5–10 minutes.

3. The corneal flap is repositioned and will heal itself quickly, so no stitches are required. Many patients report improvement in vision within 1–2 days.

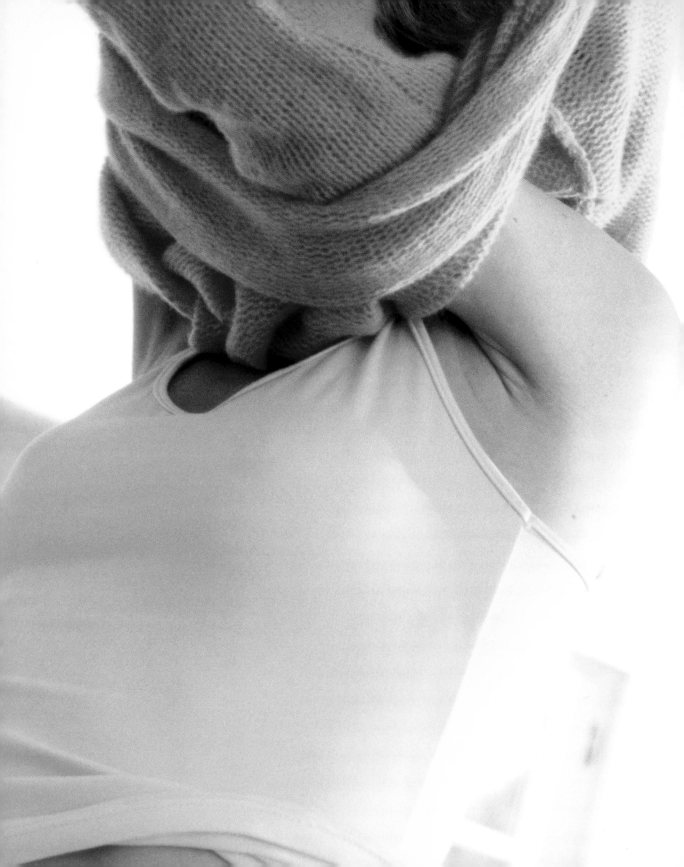

middle

In terms of overall body shape, most women know that there's no greater asset than a smooth, shapely torso. A flat stomach means that your clothes hang well and look fabulous; a firm bust gives curve and definition to your silhouette. Your shoulders, arms and hands are constantly on show every time you eat, greet and make gestures, so it's vital that they always look their best. While it's true that diet and exercise can make a serious difference to the stubborn waist area, it's also undeniable that any extra fat that settles there is notoriously hard to shift. In this section you'll find food and fitness suggestions to give you toned arms and a super-trim waist, beauty treatments to firm up your middle bits and tips about when surgery could be appropriate. Your back is covered, too, with safe, gentle exercises for strained, stressed-out backs and posture improvers to help make you strong, supple and serene.

backs to the future
Strong, supple and well-toned: if this doesn't sound like your back, it could be time to think about the way you move – and change the habits of a lifetime. Little things such as the way we sit at work, or the way we carry our handbag, can have profound effects on our bodies, leading to backache – or worse. Luckily, posture is easily corrected.

LIVE BETTER

You carry more tension in your back than in any other area of your body. While regular massages help ease stress levels and soothe aching muscles, it's important to remember that much of that tension is caused by bad posture.

But what is posture? The first thing to remember is that posture doesn't exist in isolation. It doesn't involve one set position that you should try and maintain all day. Rather, it's a dynamic, moving framework, constantly adapting and adjusting, depending on the forces it's exposed to – gravity being the main culprit.

The 'office' position causes many problems with back tension. Our spines crave freedom and balance, yet we sit slumped forward at our desks for hours at a time. This causes the hip muscles to shorten and the back muscles to lengthen, and the result is a curved spine that not only looks ungainly, but can also lead to back pain and breathing problems and eventually a condition called kyphosis – exaggerated forward bending of the spine.

To sit properly, good balance is key. Feet should be flat to the floor, knees slightly apart, your spine elongated as if someone was pulling you up by the hair and your abdominal muscles pulled in slightly. It shouldn't feel like an effort – your limbs should be soft, not tensed – but it might feel like hard work at first, as you'll more than likely have got used to some near-imperceptible tilts and twists that feel 'normal', and therefore comfortable. A small cushion placed in the small of your back can help support your back and remind you to persevere with your new endeavour to correct your position.

The same principle of a balanced body combined with evenly distributed weight and an absence of tension in the muscles applies to your standing position, too – although it's more likely to be a question of your walking posture, because few of us stand still for long periods of time. As you walk, your feet should be straight in front of you (not turned out to the sides – this can cause your hip and leg muscles to twist) and your arms should swing naturally in time to your steps. Think yourself light and springy – no mean feat when you're rushing round or exhausted, but one thing that could help is wearing special shock-absorbing inner soles.

When it comes to sleeping, experts now believe those ultra-hard, 'orthopaedic' beds may do you more harm than good – better to have a firm-ish bed that still has some 'give'. Ideally, you should sleep on your side (either one is fine) to release your spine. Sleeping on your back or front can cause tension in the lower back.

Finally, don't expect to transform yourself from hunched hedgehog to graceful swan overnight. Remember that it's not always possible to alter bad posture dramatically, but just being aware of any problems is a huge step forward.

EXERCISE BETTER

Strengthening your back doesn't mean barging into the gym and picking up the heaviest weights – it's far better to use lighter weights and do more repetitions. This will slowly strengthen your back and abdominal muscles, giving shape to muscles and creating that sought-after definition. As with any strengthening exercises, if your back starts aching, stop immediately. You can do damage to the muscles and other soft tissues of the back by lifting too much weight or lifting it in the wrong way.

Besides weight training, normal aerobic exercise is also excellent for achieving and maintaining a healthy back. Associated weight loss will, of course, help your back to look fitter and more toned. Getting your circulation pumping leads to healthier joints and vertebrae. Gentle exercise and stretching can also relieve the muscle tension that often settles in the back. Walking is particularly good for the back because it provides good aerobic exercise without putting too much strain on the back (although softer, grassy surfaces are better than roads). You could also try cycling, and especially swimming, which is strengthening yet easy on the back because the water takes away some of the strain provided by gravity. Keep your head close to the water, though, or you could end up straining your neck as you improve your back.

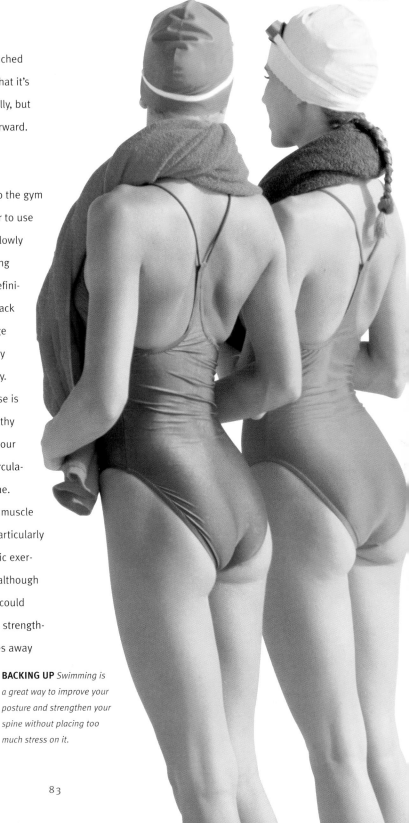

BACKING UP *Swimming is a great way to improve your posture and strengthen your spine without placing too much stress on it.*

A SHAPELIER BACK

✳ **WE** spend ages in the gym trying to sculpt our legs, arms and torsos, but the 'out of sight, out of mind' rule means we almost always overlook our backs. Try these exercises to achieve a firmer, more well-defined back.

The ideal back has a 'V' shape – strong, broad shoulders, tapering down to a trim waistline. For this, you need to concentrate on building up the latissimus dorsi, the rhomboids and the trapezius muscles. When you're performing back-strengthening exercises, try and keep your back straight, and your abdominal muscles pulled in. This gives you a firm central 'core' to work with. Currently, one of the biggest fitness crazes is for 'core' training. This means concentrating on the central 'trunk' of the body.

1. Standing curl for flexibility

Stand up straight, with your knees soft and arms hanging by your sides. Tuck your chin into your chest and, starting at the nape of your neck, slowly curl your body forward, bit by bit, until your whole spine is curled over and your arms are hanging loosely above your feet. Gently stretching your arms forward will further increase the stretch across your shoulders. Rest there for a few seconds and then begin to unfurl, taking as much time as you did to curl up in the first place.

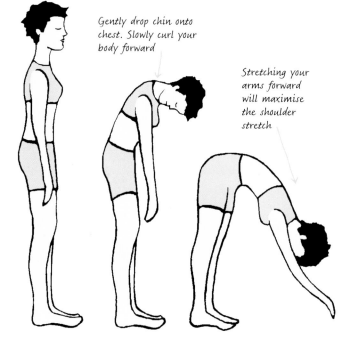

Gently drop chin onto chest. Slowly curl your body forward

Stretching your arms forward will maximise the shoulder stretch

2. Dorsal raise for lower back strength

Lie face down on the floor with your arms and legs stretched. Raise your left arm and your right leg. Keep them straight and hold for several seconds. Gently them back down to the floor and swap sides so th now raise your right arm and your left leg.
REPEAT Five times, ideally five times a week.

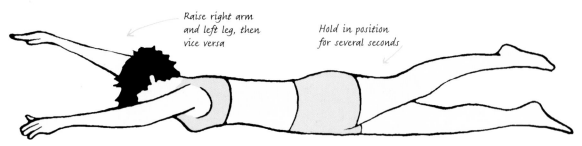

Raise right arm and left leg, then vice versa

Hold in position for several seconds

3. Extensor muscles stretch for a shapely lower back

Kneel on all fours with the palms of your hands flat to the floor. Try and keep your back straight and your abdominal muscles tight. Slowly bring one knee forward towards your head, hold for a few moments, then gently extend the same leg backwards so that it is fully extended, leg slightly raised, behind you. Hold again for a few moments. **REPEAT Five times with the same leg, then swap to the other side.**

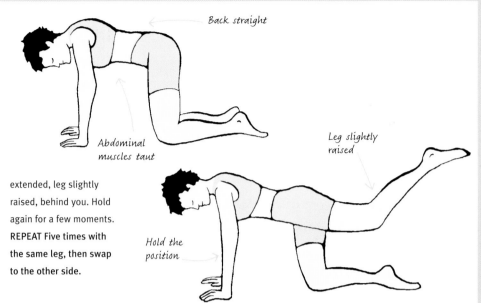

Back straight

Abdominal muscles taut

Leg slightly raised

Hold the position

4. Back raises for a toned upper back

Lie flat, face down on the floor. Your arms should be stretched out to the sides, with your elbows at right angles and your palms down, pointing forwards. Slowly raise your head, shoulders and arms off the floor – just a couple of inches will be enough. Now, slowly press your shoulder blades together and hold for a moment. Slowly lower yourself back down to the floor and rest for a moment, then repeat ten times.

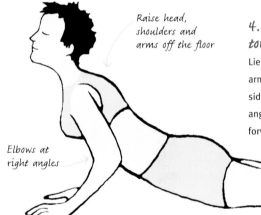

Raise head, shoulders and arms off the floor

Elbows at right angles

Yoga back rock

After exercising, relieve pressure on your back by gently massaging it, using the floor to help. Lie down on your back and bring your knees up to your stomach, hugging them with your arms. Once you have found a comfortable position, gently roll slightly to one side and then back over to the other. Rocking slowly from side to side like this for a few minutes will keep your spine warm and relaxed.

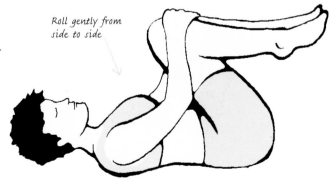

Roll gently from side to side

ease my pain

Back pain is awful – and incredibly common, too. What exactly goes wrong? Can we prevent it, and how can we make it better? Taking the best elements from conventional medicine and alternative therapies, help is at hand for bad backs – simply choose the treatment that's right for you.

PREVENTING AND TREATING PAIN

There is no doubt that, in the long term, the most crucial ways to prevent back problems are keeping fit and shedding excess weight. One of the most common forms of back pain is a generalised ache that comes from spine misalignment, often caused by carrying around those extra pounds. Age is another factor. You can't prevent the march of time, but you can make sure you're prepared for it with good exercise and dietary habits.

If you get a sudden back pain, though, there are a few immediate things to bear in mind. Contrary to popular belief, taking to your bed for a week probably isn't going to help. For a start, a sagging mattress may have contributed to the problem in the first place, and secondly, getting on the move again – however gently – stops your muscles and joints becoming weaker and will give you a more positive outlook, too. If the pain is bad, you should of course rest in a comfortable position – but don't forget this might be anything from standing or kneeling to lying on your side. When you do go to bed, sleep on your side, bending your knees, with a pillow propped between them to straighten the spinal column while you sleep. Temperature-changers such as ice packs or hot water bottles can also work. Start with a cold compress for the first couple of days, then switch to a warm one – a lavender-laced one would be even better.

TREATMENTS – WHAT YOU NEED TO KNOW

OSTEOPATHY It's hard to know how to categorise osteopathy – it's part art, part science and part treatment. It's centred around the idea that the body has the ability to keep itself in a state of optimal balance and fire up its own healing processes, so an osteopath will try and relieve pain and realign your body through massage, manipulation and gentle stretching. Osteopathy is most often used to treat generalised complaints where the cause of the problem is not completely understood, or where the pain is having a knock-on effect on other parts of the body. A pain in your foot, for example, might have a knock-on effect on your back and even your head, causing pain there, too. The principle is that your body's musculo-skeletal framework (your joints and muscles) is interdependent with the functions that it carries out: you need your joints and muscles to move, for example, but you need to move in order to keep them functional. Since so much of osteopathy depends on manual diagnosis and manual treatment, results can vary from practitioner to practitioner. Make sure you're happy with yours – all back therapies work much better when the patient is relaxed.

CHIROPRACTIC is a form of therapy that evolved from osteopathy. Where they differ is that osteopathy works on the whole body, whereas chiropractic considers the spinal column and the nerves that radiate from it the 'root' of most problems, even those in parts of the body far distant from the back. You'd be referred to a chiropractor by your doctor if tests or X-rays showed that your back pain was being caused by 'trapped' or dislodged vertebrae – often after a specific event like a car crash or sports injury. A chiropractor carries out spinal 'adjustments' by applying a high velocity, short lever arm 'thrust' to each of the affected vertebrae. This releases a mixture of gases – oxygen, nitrogen and carbon dioxide – that relieve joint pressure. Sometimes an audible 'click' can be heard as the vertebrae pop back into place. The treatment can feel mildly uncomfortable at the time, especially if your muscles are not completely relaxed. In an uncomplicated case, regular treatments can solve the problem in as little as four to six weeks.

ROLFING® can not only treat injuries, but is also used by dancers, athletes and musicians to improve their performance. It is useful for women preparing for pregnancy and labour. Unlike osteopathy and chiropractic, which work with the musculo-skeletal system, Rolfing® works by manipulating the body's superficial layers – ligaments and tendons and the deep, connective fibres that make up the fascia, a layer lying between the skin and the muscles – to stretch and realign them. The therapist guides the patient in stretching and rebalancing movements, manipulating the connective tissues as they go. As with other back treatment methods, the sensation can be painful before it is exhilarating. Though Rolfing® has been around since the 1930s, there are only around 1,200 practitioners worldwide, all of whom must have been trained by the Rolf® Institute.

Back pain glossary

Slipped disc common name for the painful condition in which one of the spongy, shock-absorbing pads (intervertebral disc) between the spinal vertebrae protrudes, causing swelling and pressure on one or more nerves of the spine; also called herniated or prolapsed disc.

Sciatica pain radiating from the buttock to lower leg, the pathway of the sciatic nerve, often caused by a disc pressing on the nerve at its spinal origin.

Inflammatory joint disease one of a number of conditions in which chronic swelling of joints causes pain and limits movement. Among those that affect the back are osteoarthritis and ankylosing spondilitis.

Osteoarthritis pain and swelling caused by 'wear and tear' on the cartilage separating the bones that form a joint; associated with ageing and more common in women than in men.

Osteoporosis weakening of bones due to loss of density associated with ageing, especially in women after menopause; may cause fractures of the vertebrae, which may result in back pain.

AND RELAX...

Even more common than acute back pain is the throbbing, grumbling backache that affects most of us at one time or another and is mostly caused by stress, tiredness and bad posture. But with a good massage, help is always at hand.

When we ask for a massage, most of us are concerned about relieving the tension in our back. The back is the largest expanse in your body, and bears the brunt of much of your stress, but when it comes to relieving that strain, a massage therapist can really make a difference. Long, sweeping strokes (effleurage) will help iron out knots caused by tension, bad posture or – in some cases – injuries.

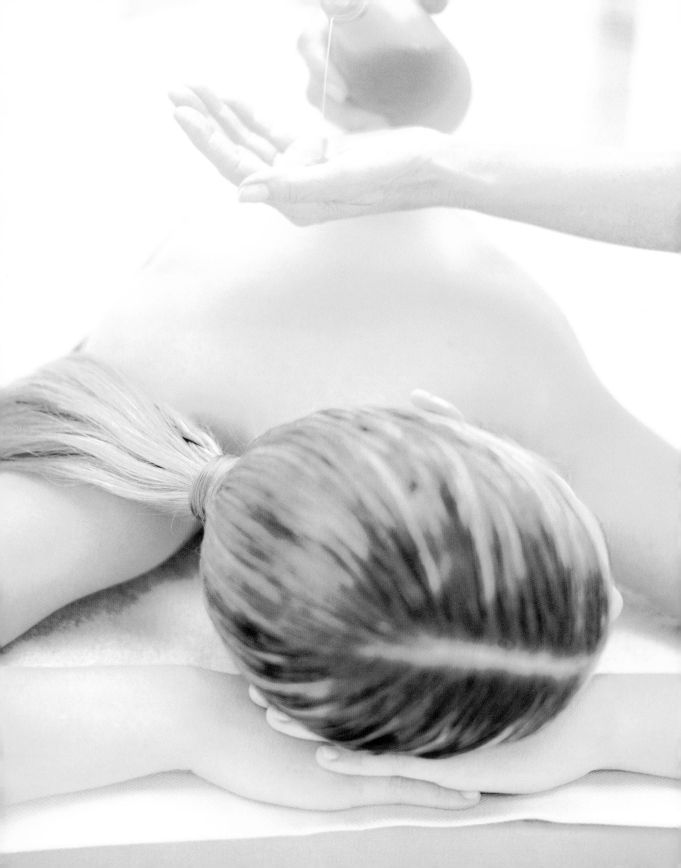

TISSUE THERAPY

Scientifically, what massage should do is normalise tissue. The massage strokes press against the soft tissue, smoothing out areas where it has become bunched up so that the blood supply can move around more easily, stimulating nerves and keeping the tissue in good condition. The most common form of massage is Swedish massage, which combines effleurage with petrissage (kneading movements), friction (deep circular movements over joints) and percussion (drumming movements to stimulate circulation). Deep tissue massage is its more thorough relation, and is excellent for chronic fatigue and aching back muscles.

If you're suffering with back problems, you need to find out if you're experiencing a localised pain or a general ache. The former is not something massage is designed to help; indeed, you could end up making things worse. The latter is a prime candidate for massage – however, it's sometimes difficult to distinguish between the two. In either case, your therapist can help you, and there will usually be a way of tailoring your treatment to avoid the questionable areas. You may have to avoid having a massage if you're pregnant (although many spas now offer special pregnancy massages), have had chemotherapy or radiation treatment, or are suffering from a skin condition, broken bones or varicose veins.

TARGETED STRESS RELIEF

For backs that ache through stress, consider one of the massages that have physical and mental benefits in equal parts. In some disciplines, physically removing the obstacles to an effective blood flow is inextricably linked to mentally eliminating blockages in your energy flow. Shiatsu, acupressure, Thai, Chinese and Ayurvedic massage systems fall into this category. Each involves the usual sweeping and circular massage movements, but uses a slightly different set of 'energy centres' as its framework.

If your aching back is caused by bad posture, a massage can help to temporarily relieve the symptoms, but it might be worth considering a system that encourages good movement, such as the Alexander Technique, which teaches you how to move in a way that complements your muscles.

Find a therapist who is either licensed or qualified by a reputable organisation such as the British Massage Therapy Council. Many of the larger beauty companies also have their own stringent training regimes, so choosing a day spa offering treatments by one of these is also a fairly safe bet.

LOVE YOUR BACK – SURGICAL OPTIONS

Many women, who have been pleased with the effects that microdermabrasion can have on facial acne scars (*see page 54*) are trying it out on their backs, too. It takes longer (simply because of the larger surface area) and can therefore be more expensive, and the effects won't be permanent, but scars can fade with repeated treatments.

For sun damage, pigmentation and more severe acne scars, dermabrasion (which uses a wheel-shaped object to remove several layers of skin at once) is sometimes recommended, but the results are not generally very effective and there is also a fairly high risk of scar formation from the treatment itself. 'For sun damage, most surgeons prefer you to take a course of topical retinoic acid and hydroquinone and combine this with a chemical peel,' says Nick Percival, Consultant Plastic Surgeon, Charing Cross Hospital, London.

healthy chest

Sore, swollen and tender breasts impact on your mood, your wardrobe – your whole lifestyle in fact. But are you really doing everything you possibly can to keep breast tenderness at bay? It's not always a question of grinning and bearing it. Taking into account such factors as your age, your hormones and your menstrual cycle, you may find that there are certain foods and herbs in nature's storecupboard that can help to relieve the nagging pain.

TENDER LOVING CARE

If you regularly experience sore, tender or swollen breasts, you probably put it down to your hormones, or vaguely decide that you must be at some important point in your menstrual cycle. Both are probably true – but chances are your diet could be partly to blame as well. For example, women who have a fairly healthy diet, with lots of fresh fruit and vegetables, seem less prone to PMS and all its attendant misery (including stomach-ache, headaches and sore breasts) than those who snack on junk food and fizzy drinks.

If your breast soreness is due to PMS, stepping up your oil intake for a few days could be a good move. Eat nuts and oily fish to increase your levels of essential fatty acids, and take evening primrose or starflower oil for their gamma linolenic acid (GLA), both of which can help reduce inflammation. The evening primrose oil is best taken in daily supplements that may take a few months to really kick in, but advocates say its PMS-fighting effects are worth the wait. Vitamin E supplements are also good for breast soreness – both taken internally and gently massaged straight into the tender areas. Premenstrual breast soreness is often related

to high levels of oestrogen in your bloodstream: decreasing the fat and increasing the fibre in your diet can help cause oestrogen levels to dip.

If your breast tenderness is happening at other times, this could mean that your diet is deficient in calcium and magnesium. Women approaching, experiencing or leaving behind the menopause often suffer with sore breasts, and it's no coincidence that these are also the times at which they're told to boost their intake of calcium and magnesium. In addition, watch out if you've got a particularly sweet tooth – eating large quantities of sugary foods can cause magnesium levels to dip. Make sure you eat plenty of wholewheat cereal, avocados, almonds, potatoes, pulses and fish for magnesium and take a calcium supplement (it's quite difficult to get your full daily quota of calcium from your diet).

Another reason why it could be better to take a calcium supplement than stock up on dairy is the opinion of some people that reducing one's intake of dairy products actually helps in the fight against breast cancer. The theory goes that the reason why breast and prostate cancers are much rarer in China and Japan than they are in the West is because of the difference between the two diets. What exactly makes those Eastern immune systems so much healthier is yet to be proven conclusively, but the lack of dairy products in Eastern diets compared to those in the West is thought to play a major part.

Where there's breast tenderness, there's often also water retention. Fluid gets trapped in the fatty parts of the breasts, making them swell and feel painful. Combat this by reducing the amount of salt in your diet and eating potassium-rich foods that will balance the sodium (and therefore reduce the level of retained fluid) in your body. Good sources of potassium are mushrooms, bananas and

tomatoes. Keep caffeine – in fact, all diuretics – to a minimum, too. Hot drinks can be comforting, especially when you've got PMS, but if you like herb teas, try and stick to them instead of ordinary tea or coffee. Camomile and rosehip tea are both soothing.

HERBS TO HELP

Nature's own medicine cabinet contains a few good things to help relieve sore breasts. A full body massage with geranium essential oil, or a few drops of the oil in your bath, is said to help ease fluid retention, and would be particularly effective a few days before your period. Topical application of St John's Wort oil, a fabulous natural pain reliever that can actually penetrate nerve endings, can also help – smooth this gently into your breasts.

Evening primrose oil, as we've seen, is also fantastic for PMS, either taken orally in capsule form or massaged straight into the skin (it smells so delicious that it also makes a wonderful bath oil) and borage oil can also reduce tenderness. Ginseng is also fantastic for decreasing fluid retention and generally giving yourself a bit of a vitality boost into the bargain. You can buy ginseng tablets, but its leaves also make a delicious cup of tea – just the thing for those achy, 'down' days.

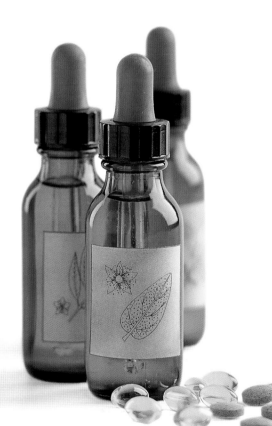

ESSENTIAL REMEDIES
To relieve soreness, add some essential oils, such as evening primrose or borage, to your bath or massage blend.

keeping abreast

Are your breasts beginning to lose their elasticity? Don't grab the telephone book and search under 'S' for surgeon...think 'E' for exercise instead. You won't gain a cup size, but there are certain exercises that you can do to improve the shape and tone of your breasts.

THE RIGHT APPROACH

Is it really possible to increase the size of your bust just by doing exercise? Yes and no. Because there's no muscle actually in your breasts, they won't respond to strength training – end of story. However, you can tone up the pectoral muscles that lie directly beneath the breasts, and increase your upper body mass.

Good posture can also help. Keep your shoulders set back (not so that you arch your back in the style of those clichéd glamour models – that would be a little obvious!) and also keep them low, so that you carry your weight low down in your back, rather than in the middle.

Remember that the pectoral muscles are very small. No matter how much training you do, you're never going to develop huge, outwardly curving mounds beneath your breasts to propel them outwards. The only way to do that is with implants, and that's another story (involving a general anaesthetic and a large pile of cash). Normally, implants will never give you a cleavage (unless they are very large ones), which is something muscle-boosting exercises should certainly be able to offer.

Remember that breast exercises are dependent on how big your breasts are – the heavier they are, the harder the muscles will have to work and the smaller the effect is likely to be. If they are saggy to begin with, gravity is on their side, so again, it's hard for the pectoral muscles to make a difference. Resistance exercises that will give the appearance of larger breasts are more about maintenance than correction, so the rule is to start early and practise regularly – a minimum of three times a week would be ideal.

To begin with, try a push-up – but slightly modified so that you're focusing on the chest area, not on your abdominals (though hopefully it should also benefit them, too – isn't exercise great?). Begin by lying face down on the floor, with your palms flat and your toes pointing away from you, just as you would normally for a push-up. The important thing is that instead of pushing your whole body up, you need to keep your knees flat to the floor and push up gently with your hands, focusing on your chest and feeling your chest muscles working. Rest for a moment and repeat ten times. For a less strenuous exercise, stand up straight, arms out to the side. Make circles in the air, about 50 cm (20 inches) in diameter, first one way, then the other. Repeat eight times.

If you go to the gym or have access to free weights, another good exercise is the chest press. Lie on your back on a bench, keeping your legs soft but your abdominals tight and take a weight in each hand. The tops of your arms should be touching the bench, but your elbows will be at 90 degrees so that the weights are resting above you, at either side of your head. Slowly stretch your arms upwards until they are nearly locked, pause, then return to the 'resting' position (with the tops of your arms on the bench).

THE RIGHT EQUIPMENT

Some conventional forms of exercise, such as swimming, are fabulous for the breasts – water gives a natural support and the gentle repetitive motion of breast stroke helps to enhance curves. It doesn't take a genius to work out why others, such as running and aerobics classes (anything that involves springing up and then coming back down) are not so chest friendly. How much lasting damage you can do is open to debate. Some experts say that sporty women will stretch and damage ligaments and other breast tissues, and even cite examples of collarbones breaking because of the sudden movement of very heavy breasts. Others argue that with a properly fitting bra, it should be possible for women to play sport without worrying about lasting damage. The key phrase here, though, is 'properly fitting'. Sports bras are relatively new on the market and vary in their effectiveness: even the best ones will give only around 20 per cent more protection than a normal, well-fitting bra.

However, newer designs harness each breast separately, with reinforced shoulders to reduce 'shock' caused by jumping around. They often have a 'racer' back to prevent straps slipping. They're generally considered a wise investment, particularly for larger breasted women. Once you've got the right bra, it's all down to good fitness posture. When you run, propel yourself forward all the way down from your ankles, chest slightly forward. Never bend from the waist.

Sports bras – what to look for

LARGE breasts and energetic workouts do not a breast-friendly combination make, but whatever your cup size, every woman who works out regularly should invest in a good sports bra. Vigorous activity will put stress on the breast tissue, so a sports bra must provide adequate support as well as being comfortable and ventilated. Look for the following qualities.

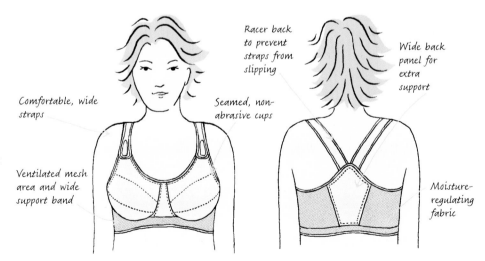

Comfortable, wide straps

Ventilated mesh area and wide support band

Racer back to prevent straps from slipping

Seamed, non-abrasive cups

Wide back panel for extra support

Moisture-regulating fabric

93

beauty or bust

Exercises aren't working. Bras aren't working. You can't face the thought of surgery. Is there a miracle cream that can help? Before you spend the money, find out what the latest products can do, and whether a salon treatment could help.

BREAST SCEPTICS

For all that we complain about the size, shape, firmness, fullness, tone, texture and even colour of our breasts, in terms of our beauty routine, we tend to pay them very little attention – it's enough for most of us to smooth a bit of body lotion over them in the mornings. Why this should be is a very interesting question. Maybe we presume that, short of surgery, a bra is the best way to transform the shape of our breasts. Perhaps it's also that we're naturally sceptical about the claims of bust-firming creams and lotions – it does seem incredible that a moisturiser, however high-tech it may be, should be able to defy gravity. It could also be that we realise that beauty solutions to sagging breasts will take time and effort to achieve – commodities that, with our hectic lives, we'd rather spend doing other things.

SHORT CUTS FOR BETTER BREASTS

If time is your biggest obstacle, perhaps booking in for a bust-firming salon treatment could be your best bet. The results won't be long-lasting – a couple of days at most – but might give you an extra 'lift' in time for a special night out. Be warned, though – you won't get the usual sleep-inducing massage and relaxing oils that you might associate with beauty salons. These treatments are usually all about toning the underlying muscles and eliminating water retention with an icy-cold jet of water that's aimed at each breast for several minutes.

FIRM FRIENDS *For those who don't want to go down the surgical route, try some of the latest breast-boosting treatments.*

A nice massage may follow with stimulating essential oils so that you don't leave the salon in too much of a state of shock. Make a note of the oils they're using so you can try the same thing at home, or choose from stimulating juniper, rosemary or ylang-ylang essential oils. Massage itself will not help increase bust size, but it does have other benefits for your breasts. For example, a massage that helps drain the lymphatic system may also, over time, help reduce pigmentation marks on the bust and nipple.

Links are also currently being made between chronically poor breast drainage and the risk of breast cancer. Anything that inhibits the lymph system, such as a too-tight bra or wearing a bra for overly long periods of time, is thought to increase the risk, while breast massage can decrease it. You can self-massage your breasts: general kneading, rubbing and squeezing strokes will increase blood and lymph flow to the breast. Start at the nipple and work outwards, and remember to use only light to moderate pressure to avoid hurting or bruising this most sensitive of areas.

SHORT-TERM SOLUTIONS

For firmer breasts, the scary-sounding 'suction' technique is one step on from hydrotherapy. For this procedure, a cone-shaped 'plunger' is attached to the breast, then air is pumped out, encouraging breast tissue to swell and also sit high on the front of the breast. It's not so much painful as just mildly disconcerting, and again, the effects will last for only a couple of days. Watch this space, though – scientists are currently working on a futuristic 'booster' bra with tiny computer-controlled vacuums inside the two bra 'pockets'!

Another treatment that underdeveloped women sometimes turn to is hypnotherapy. There's no medical evidence for its efficacy, just anecdotal accounts that hypnotherapy can make a difference to the size of your breasts. It's fair to say that the success rates do not match those for, say, giving up smoking or conquering phobias, simply because these latter treatments deal with states of mind rather than physical attributes. Having said that, combined with exercise and beauty treatments, it may have an effect and the only way to know is to try – but be wary of laying out large sums of money up front (no pun intended).

So-called 'bra in a jar' treatments (which you apply yourself) are similar to cellulite creams – they need applying regularly, usually every morning and evening, if you're to see the cumulative effect, which manufacturers usually claim will take around six weeks. They offer varying degrees of space-age technology and impressive-sounding results, but in the main, if they work at all, they do so by stimulating circulation and causing slight and transitory swelling. Smaller breasts are more likely to show an improvement because they have less of a fight on their hands with gravity!

From a purely aesthetic point of view, you could consider good old-fashioned padding. This is no longer a question of stuffing some tissues into your cups. The new pads are curved, flesh-coloured and squishy – just like the real things, in fact. In the fashion industry, they are often used by models on shoots and are generally referred to as 'chicken fillets' because of their startling resemblance to raw poultry. When it comes to more revealing outfits, no female celebrity is complete without her TitTape™ – skin-friendly double-sided sticky tape that holds the breasts in place.

the right curves
Since breast augmentation began thirty years ago, it has never been far from controversy. Sorting the essential facts from the general furore is vital with any surgery, but especially when it's something so close to your heart....

TAKING THE SURGICAL ROUTE

Breasts are associated with femininity, and many women who are unhappy with the size or shape of theirs feel less 'womanly' as a result. While no-one should see breast augmentation as a 'quick fix' or magic key to instant desirability, there's no doubt that it's helped countless women feel better about themselves.

It's not always simply about magnifying what nature gave you, either. Some women have underdeveloped breasts, some have seen their breast size decrease after pregnancy or weight loss and some have asymmetrical breasts that they want to even out. Augmentation mammaplasty can help with all of these problems. Unless you're having very large implants, one thing it can't do is create a cleavage, but most women find that with their newly enhanced shape, all it takes is a push-up bra to achieve the desired effect.

'It's not possible for surgeons to predict how breast implants will "take" – in the same way that people form different types of scars on the skin's surface, they can also react differently to foreign substances internally, too.'
Nick Percival, Consultant Plastic Surgeon, Charing Cross Hospital, London

Once you've decided on surgery, your chest, heart and blood will all be examined, and you may also be given a mammogram (X-ray of the breast tissue). Contrary to widely held belief, it does not necessarily follow that breast implants will make it more difficult to have mammograms in the future. As we'll see, implants are placed either behind the breast or behind the muscle underneath the breast, and therefore the breast tissue itself can be easily visualised. The pre-operative mammogram is to detect any problems.

The operation is performed under general anaesthetic or local anaesthesia with a sedative. It's usually a day case, but you may be kept in overnight if there's no-one to look after you in the first forty-eight hours. You can't eat for at least six hours before the operation. Where the incision will be made largely depends on your surgeon: some work through incisions in the curve beneath the breast (inframammary location), others the nipple (the periareolar approach) and others may make incisions in the armpit (the axillary approach) as this is thought to be the least conspicuous.

Depending on how thin you are, the implant will then be placed either beneath the breast tissue or deeper in, beneath the pectoralis major muscle that sits underneath the breast – if your breasts are small and you have a slight frame, the implant may be too noticeable if it's close to the surface, so it is 'buried' beneath the muscle tissue.

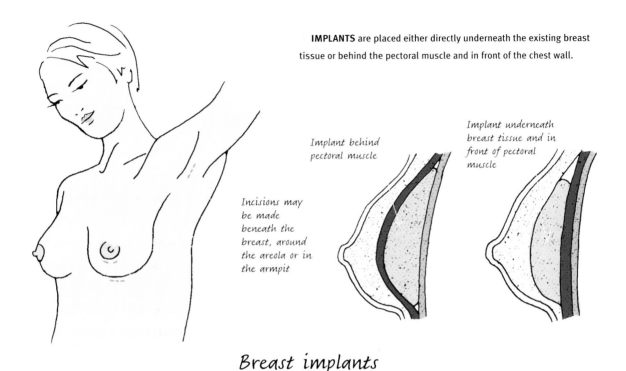

IMPLANTS are placed either directly underneath the existing breast tissue or behind the pectoral muscle and in front of the chest wall.

Implant behind pectoral muscle

Implant underneath breast tissue and in front of pectoral muscle

Incisions may be made beneath the breast, around the areola or in the armpit

Breast implants

WHICH IMPLANT?

Silicone implants are still used throughout much of Europe. but in the United States implants are now most commonly made from saline (salt water). There is a small risk of implants leaking once they've been inserted; if your breast shrinks after surgery, this could be the reason, so you must have it checked out. Saline implants are thought to be safe because the salt water will be easily absorbed by the body's tissues, but silicone gives a more natural-looking appearance. There has been a big scare about connections between silicone and breast and autoimmune disease, but no links have been found. It's also important to remember that instances of implant leakage have been reduced – though not entirely eliminated – with the advent of the

modern, thicker-walled implants. Whatever type of implant you are considering or have had, it's important to have them checked annually and replaced every ten years – so be aware that implants constitute a continuing cost commitment.

THE ROAD TO RECOVERY

The most common complications associated with the operation are excessive bleeding during and after the operation (some surgeons will insert a drain for the first twenty-four hours after the operation) and the formation of a hard wall of tissue around the implant (known as capsular contracture). It can cause firm, painful and misshapen breasts, and the implants have to be removed. It's not

what a waist

Shaving inches off your middle makes your clothes fit better and your curves more shapely – just ask the corset-wearing ladies of the 18th century. Thank goodness we've got a modern alternative to help us to achieve a slimmer-looking body.

WAIST REMOVAL

Lipoplasty is great for slimming hips and thighs, but when it comes to trimming our waist, things aren't that simple. For a start, it's hard to talk about the waist in isolation. The appearance of your waist is dependent not only on the amount of fat stored around your middle (and the amount of fat inside the abdominal cavity – above the navel – that cannot be treated with lipoplasty), but also on the relative size of your chest and hips. (Large hips, though perhaps not desirable in themselves, will give the illusion of a trimmer waist and vice versa.)

For this reason, when lipoplasty is used to create a shapelier waist, it's always planned in relation to other parts of the body, particularly the hips and thighs – they will not all be operated on at the same time, but might be considered for follow-up procedures. When surgeons talk about 'narrower waist lipoplasty', they're actually referring to three places – the abdomen, flanks and under-the-bra area. These three can be worked on together.

TUMMY TUCK (ABDOMINOPLASTY)

The stubborn layer of fat that sits around the waistline gets harder and harder to shift as we get older. Sometimes it seems as if no amount of exercise can make any difference (in some cases, it won't – an abdominal 'bulge' can be an inherited condition and if your weight is 'middle-age spread' it can be similarly difficult to budge without surgery). Also, if you were left with 'surplus' skin following weight loss or pregnancy, there's precious little you can do to shift it on your own – a 'tummy tuck' could be the answer you are looking for.

A tummy tuck works in two ways: first, it firms, then it flattens. The 'firming' is done by removing the unwanted fat and tightening the underlying abdominal muscles (sometimes the muscles can also be pushed together slightly so the new look is more natural). The 'flattening' is done by reducing the amount of skin on top of these muscles, so that the remaining skin is stretched tighter, giving a smoother look. This part can often help diminish the appearance of stretch marks, too, if they're cut off at the same time. The skin is lifted away from the tissue at the bra area, then pulled all the way down towards the groin. There's also a partial technique called a 'mini tummy tuck' that concentrates solely on fat that's collected below the navel. In both cases, excess skin is removed and the shortened piece sewn back into place. This can be done by making just one incision, usually in a horizontal line within the top of the pubic area, which means it should be well camouflaged, although sometimes it is extended up towards the hip bones at each side (this can easily be hidden by underwear).

The operation requires a general anaesthetic and, in the same way as 'normal' lipoplasty, it contains all the associated surgical risks such as swelling, bruising, infection and scarring (*see pages 26–27*). More specifically, when fat is removed by lipoplasty, there's a certain amount of 'redistribution' of the fat that's left. This means that although lipoplasty may let you trim pounds from the 'spare tyre' around your middle, the fat that's left after the surgery may 'spread out' slightly, so that although you're now leaner round the middle, you still haven't got a trim, curvaceous waist. The biggest advantage is that, barring excessive weight gain, your tummy should stay flatter for years to come.

ABDOMINAL ETCHING

Some people are never happy. A washboard-flat stomach not enough? Want that super-realistic muscle definition that will convince everyone you've been doing 100 abdominal crunches a day? Thank goodness the surgeons are one step ahead of you. Small-volume lipoplasty can now be used to hoover up any layers of fat that are sitting directly over your abdominal muscles so that the muscles can show through, creating that lean, toned 'rippled' effect. (It's almost always performed on men, but some athletic women have been requesting it, too.) Of course, it goes without saying that if you exercise regularly, your muscles will be bigger and have a better chance of showing up.

Abdominoplasty

TUMMY TUCK (abdominoplasty) procedures differ slightly, depending on individual requirements. An incision is made around the navel and then a new opening is cut when the skin is pulled down.

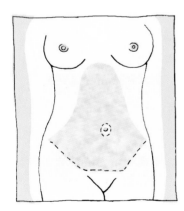
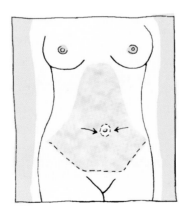
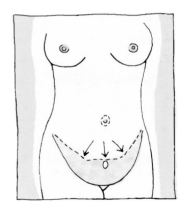

Incisions are made just below the 'bikini line' and around the navel. Skin is then lifted away from the abdominal wall (shaded).

Secondly, the underlying tissue and muscles are pulled together and stitched into a new position to create a firm abdominal wall.

Excess skin is removed and the remaining skin pulled down towards the pubic area. A new opening is cut for the navel.

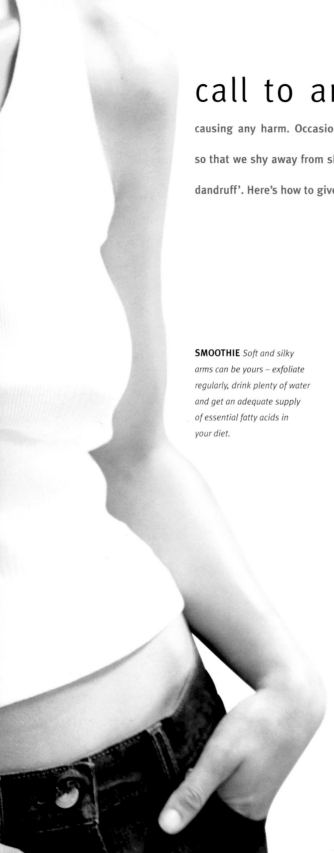

call to arms

Most of the time arms swing along nicely, not causing any harm. Occasionally, though, they get dry and scaly, sometimes so much so that we shy away from skimpy tops for fear of drawing attention to this horrible 'arm dandruff'. Here's how to give dry skin the elbow, naturally.

SMOOTHIE *Soft and silky arms can be yours – exfoliate regularly, drink plenty of water and get an adequate supply of essential fatty acids in your diet.*

EATING FOR TWO

Surprise, surprise – when it comes to our arms, dry, scaly skin is the most common complaint. What's not so obvious is that dry skin sufferers often have trouble digesting fats effectively: it might be that they're consuming fewer essential fatty acids than they need to, or it may be that they're lacking in related nutrients. Lack of vitamin A and the B vitamins, for example, may also hinder the EFA absorption process. Cell-renewing vitamin A can also help eradicate that other strange arm condition so many of us often notice: those funny little white pimples around the tops of our arms. These are often caused by dead skin cell build-up, so as well as exfoliating regularly and drinking lots of water, a diet of fresh antioxidant vegetables (such as green, leafy ones) can keep cells ticking over properly.

ESSENTIAL THERAPY

There are different essential fatty acids, with different uses in the body. The two main groups are the alpha-linolenic acid group (also known as the LNA or Omega 3 group) and the linoleic acid group (LA or Omega 6 group). Researchers are still learning about how the body uses these substances, but this much is known: they seem to have a beneficial effect on cholesterol and triglyceride levels in the blood, making them a good bet for reducing the risk of heart disease. Both are used by the brain. Omega 6 seems to play a role in the immune system. They seem to work best when they are present in equal amounts, but the typical Western diet contains twenty times more Omega 6 than Omega 3 oils, so you should concentrate on fish, tofu and nuts, and go easy on vegetable oils. Latest research suggests that Omega 3 could play an important part in weight loss: the theory goes that it can help regulate blood sugar levels, so it could potentially work as a natural appetite suppressant. Be careful when using the foods as oils, though: it's easy for EFA levels to diminish when the oils are extracted – especially if they're exposed to heat, light or air. Make sure the variety you buy is cold-pressed, oxygen-free and kept in a dark bottle. Once opened, keep it in the refrigerator.

If you're concerned about the skin on your arms and suspect that your diet isn't up to scratch, it could be worth considering taking one of the supplements formulated specifically to encourage healthy skin. They boost keratin production, the protein from which skin, hair and nails are all made and maintained. There are many different varieties of healthy skin supplements – but essentially the good ones will contain all the nutrients mentioned above, plus vitamin E to soften and strengthen the skin, and often a good dose of other antioxidants to help protect it, too. Zinc is also important because it helps with cellular repair. After taking supplements for four to six weeks, most scaly skin sufferers report seeing an improvement, saying that their skin 'feels like it's been moisturised' even without body lotion.

HEATED DEBATE

As well as outer arm considerations, certain foods can present underarm problems, too. Sweat-inducing foods include marigold, thyme, garlic, onion, chives, mustard, green tea, chilli and alcohol. Perspiration itself is odourless. Any smell is the result of bacteria acting on oily substances in the sweat. Interestingly, the sweat from the underarm and pubic areas is the only sort that develops a smell. A different type of gland produces the sweat from other parts of your body, and bacteria do not colonise it. It's worth avoiding 'sweaty' foods when you know there's a high-pressure situation coming up at work, because nervousness can produce copious perspiration, often up to five times more abundant than when you are exercising or in hot weather.

Sweating is sometimes seen as the scourge of the modern, sophisticated individual, but it's important to remember that sweating is natural: it's your body's way of eliminating toxins. Every body likes to keep its tell-tale damp patches (and worse, body odour), at bay but some deodorants – those labelled 'anti-perspirant' – inhibit the sweating process so that those toxins remain in the body, effectively 'clogging up' your circulation. Aluminium-free deodorants are available from health-food shops, or to be completely new-age you could try a crystal deodorant, made of mineral salts, which works by altering the environment so it's hostile to the odour-causing bacteria. However, if you're worried that these won't be heavy-duty enough for your needs, it may be more than your deodorant you need to change: shave under your armpits regularly; wear loose, natural-fibre clothing; and wash regularly (for on-the-spot refreshening, keep a pack of deodorant wipes in your bag).

long, lean and lovely
Toned shoulders and sculpted arms make summer dressing an absolute pleasure, and they also make your upper body leaner and stronger. They take time to achieve, but rest assured it can be done – here's how.

TIME TO TONE

As with almost any other part of the body, untoned arms are more likely to be caused by excess fat than by untrained muscles – and the tops of the arms, like the hips, are flab storage sites that are particularly common to women. In the first instance, it's important to try and shift as much of this extra weight as possible – which is, of course, easier said than done. But there are subtle extra ways in which you can enhance both your everyday movements and your exercise routine to move things along. Maybe now is the time to renew your interest in gardening: all that digging, raking and weeding can do wonders for the upper arms!

Some aerobics classes can be stepped-up a gear by using free weights in some routines, and gym machines like cross trainers score a double whammy by working arms and legs at the same time. In the daytime, when you're walking briskly, try and swing your arms a little to get some momentum going. The increased aerobic exercise will benefit your whole body but the resistance work will help your arms particularly. In the gym, try and do this on the treadmill, too.

If your excuse is your ever-present bag, it could be time to break this habit, too. Rucksacks may call to mind camping trips, but you can get seriously stylish, mini ones that will leave your arms free to move (and help your spine and posture by distributing the extra weight evenly).

BICEPS, TRICEPS

If it's not so much flabby as contour-less arms that's the problem, that's when spot-treating exercise comes into its own. However, when many women start this, they notice that while the tone of their upper arms improves, the underneath just carries on jiggling around. That's because many strengthening exercises concentrate indirectly on the biceps and ignore the triceps (the two-part muscle to the front of the upper arms that help you to pull), so they're already getting a workout. For the triceps try the lat machine in the gym; you pull or push down a weighted bar that hangs from a cable. At home, just doing plain old push-ups will really help. Beware of over-working your arm muscles: they're a small muscle group and you want to stimulate, not exhaust the muscles. At first, do only between five and fifteen repetitions.

Arm exercises are one of the few types that really do benefit from investing in extra equipment, such as dumbbells (free weights) and the newer 'tubes', which are like big rubber skipping ropes. You stand with both feet on the tube and then take the ends in each hand, slowly pulling up to perform a bicep curl. Dumbbells, as opposed to barbells, are great for beginners because they allow natural movement and reduce stress on arm joints. They can also be used sitting down!

CLASS ACT

If classes are more your thing, don't assume you won't get the kind of targeted approach that your arms need. BodyPump, like an aerobics class, is done in a group, to upbeat, motivating music – but instead of jumping around frenetically and getting an aerobic workout, you use adjustable barbells to get a slower-moving, strength work-out that focuses on every major muscle group in the body.

Results can be fast, but the class works best for people who have serious amounts of muscle still to gain. If you're already pretty toned, the fact that you can only use a weight that you can lift for every movement, as opposed to lifting one from a resting position, may mean that some muscles don't get the workout they need.

Yoga classes can also give great arm workouts. In 'power yoga', you often get some aerobic benefit as well as strengthening muscles, while in more traditional styles of yoga, it's much more obvious which muscle groups are being worked on at any one time. Another great benefit of yoga is that, unlike gym-based resistance workouts, there's no capacity for building up slowly: as soon as you're ready to try a position, you often need to bear the weight of your whole body at once. There are many positions in yoga where the arms can take the majority of the body's weight, and it can quickly lengthen arms and make them more flexible into the bargain. If you have weak wrists though, you'll need to modify the exercises because full weight bearing may be a problem.

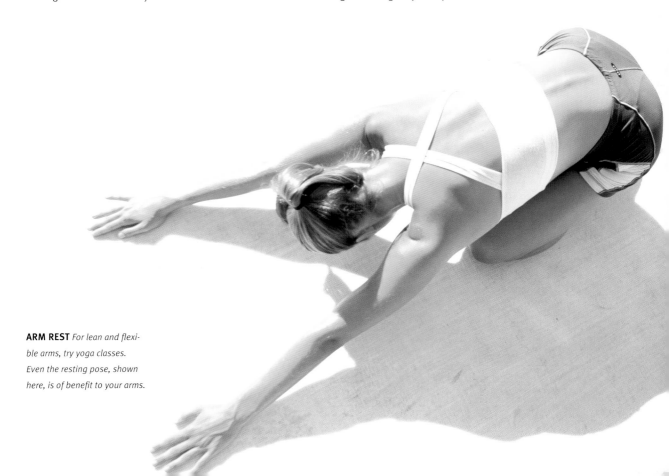

ARM REST *For lean and flexi-ble arms, try yoga classes. Even the resting pose, shown here, is of benefit to your arms.*

Arm yourself

AS WITH any exercise, it's best to keep your routine as varied as possible. This routine has been devised to work by following the exercises straight through from 1 to 6; alternatively, you can pick and choose. Remember that if it's the top of your arms you're concerned about, concentrate on exercises for your biceps, but if it's wobbly underarms, go for the tricep moves. Finally, don't overdo it: the arm muscles are small, and overworking them will cause them to shut down, not expand.

Curl arm up towards shoulder

1. Curls (for biceps)

For this you need dumbbells – two of equal weight – one in each hand. Hold them palms out in front of you and one at a time curl the arms up towards the shoulder. Begin with light weights and just ten or twelve repetitions, and increase over time. Once you're proficient, vary the exercise so that you do one set with palms out and one set with palms in, so that you work both the biceps and triceps equally.

2. Arm raises (for biceps and shoulders)

Similar to the curls in that you need two dumbbells (or two equally weighted objects such as books or bottles). Stand up straight, dumbbells by your sides, arms relaxed. Take it in turns to lift each arm straight out to the side in a nice, flowing movement. Stop when the arm is in line with the shoulder, hold, and slowly lower. Repeat ten times. That's a 'lateral' arm raise, and you can also do a 'front' arm raise by adopting the same start position except with your palms facing down, and alternately bringing each arm up in front of you until it is outstretched.

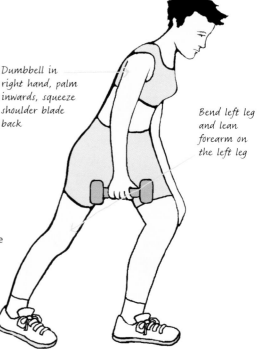

Dumbbell in right hand, palm inwards, squeeze shoulder blade back

Bend left leg and lean forearm on the left leg

3. One-arm row (for biceps, shoulders and middle back)

Put your left foot one step in front of the other. Bend the left leg and extend your right leg back as if stretching out your calf muscles. Let your left forearm lean on your left leg, and lean forwards so your left arm is taking the weight. Take a dumbbell in your right hand and let it hang down, palm inwards. Slowly squeeze your right shoulder blade back, then relax. Swap sides. REPEAT each side five times.

4. Dips (for triceps)

Sit right on the edge of a chair, so that you're comfortably balanced but your hips are over the edge. Place your palms on the chair on either side your hips, with your fingers hanging over the edge. Feet should be flat to the floor but knees soft and back comfortably straight. With your knees still bent, lower your bottom to the floor until your upper arms are parallel to the floor (keep your back straight and feet flat on the floor throughout). Then concentrate on raising yourself back up, using your upper arms as the lead. Do three sets of between ten and twenty.

Keep back as close as possible to the chair

5. Fall (for triceps and shoulders)

Stand about 3 feet (1 m) away from a wall. Fall in towards it and take the strain of your body weight in your arms. Push off from the wall to help you achieve a standing position again (this one is also good for strengthening the hands). **REPEAT ten times.**

Push away from the wall

Take the strain in your arms

6. Push-ups (triceps, shoulders and abdominals)

Push-ups are also recommended for toning the abdominal muscles – that's no surprise, since there's often a link between ab and arm exercises. This push-up is modified, however, to give the backs of the arms a turbo-charged workout, by raising the feet off the floor – either with an exercise step if you have one, or a bench, or the bottom rung of a chair. **REPEAT twenty times.**

Works the triceps, shoulders and abs

take up arms

Arms are subject to all manner of stresses and strains in the name of daily life. There's writing, typing, using telephones and calculators, reaching for things, DIY tasks, driving and of course playing sports. Don't neglect them. Love them. Keep a watchful eye on your posture and indulge with some great moisturising home treatments. Here's how.

STRONG AND HEALTHY

Tennis elbow (lateral humeral epicondylitis) is one of the most frequently diagnosed conditions in the Western world. It occurs when the tendon that attaches the forearm muscle to the elbow joint is damaged, either by overuse caused by a repetitive action in say, sport or your job or by an injury like a fall on the elbow or a bump to the arm. It's different to 'golfer's elbow' because tennis elbow involves damage to the outside (lateral) of the elbow, which is therefore where most pain is felt, while 'golfer's elbow' affects the inside (medial). Both principally produce pain in the upper arm, but it can feel stiff and tender right down to the wrist and make straightening your arm incredibly uncomfortable. Treatment involves resting the arm for the first few days, followed by a combination of physiotherapy, massage, ice packs and a non-steroidal anti-inflammatory to reduce swelling and relieve pain. If the symptoms have not disappeared in a week or two, a doctor may try cortisone injections.

There are things you can do to prevent tennis elbow. If it's the result of a sports injury, see a fitness instructor to check your posture is to blame, and perhaps even ask him or her to have a look at your equipment, too.

With tennis, for example, you can now get shock-absorbing racquets that take some of the strain away from your arm. It's also important to warm up properly. After sport, apply an ice pack to your elbow. If you don't know the cause of the problem, check your sitting posture at work or wherever you spend most time. Remember you should be looking straight ahead, not twisted round, with both feet flat to the floor. Your wrists shouldn't be resting on your keyboard but should be elevated, and frequently used items like telephones should be within easy reach.

These measures will also go some way to preventing that other scourge of the healthy arm – repetitive strain injury (RSI). The good news is that RSI is preventable, but the best course is to nip it in the bud. Pain and tingling sensations are the first early-warning signal. Try to identify the cause and stop doing whatever it is. If it is associated with activity in the workplace, bring it to the attention of your employer, who is obligated to take steps to avoid the need for the repetitive activity. It is also important to see a doctor, who will do tests to confirm the diagnosis and rule out other serious conditions, such as rheumatoid arthritis and multiple sclerosis. Do not wait until it gets so bad you cannot tolerate the pain. Treatment is usually more successful if it is started early. Non-steroidal anti-inflammatories may be prescribed, but the most important prescription is to avoid the repeated action that is responsible, and if that is not possible, take frequent breaks.

SOFT AND SILKY

As far as specific products are concerned, the arms represent one of the ever-diminishing groups of body parts that don't have their own selection of dedicated preparations. That's because the arms are served well enough by the huge array of body lotions on offer. Don't skimp on the body lotion – richness varies from product to product, but you should use at least two good dollops of body lotion for a full body application. As you're working down your arms, don't just stop at your wrists – make sure that the backs of your hands get a good moisture drink, too – and don't forget to give your elbows some attention: they can often benefit from an extra spot of primping. Slough away any scaly patches with an exfoliator (don't throw old facial scrubs away – just scoop out the last remnants and rub them into your elbows) or invest in a nail brush for the purposes of dry brushing elbows and knees – it works a treat.

The short sleeve-demanding summer makes arms a great place to wear your favourite fragrance. We move our arms around constantly, and this means that they're able to fill the air with gorgeous scents, and in any case, it's a good idea to avoid traditional alcohol-based scents during the summer because they can irritate sensitive skins and even lead to splotchy pigmentation. If your favourite fragrance doesn't have a body lotion, you can easily mix your own by putting a blob of fragrance-free moisturiser in your hands and adding a few drops of perfume. You could even experiment by doing the same thing with different essential oils according to your mood. Favourite fragrant combinations include lime and basil (for an energising effect), sandalwood and vanilla (relaxing) and rose and jasmine (sensual). Finally, if you do suffer from the occasional painful arm or elbow, keep your body lotion in the refrigerator – it will feel deliciously soothing when applied.

ESSENTIAL OILS *Add a little drop of your favourite essential oil to a fragrance-free body lotion and smooth it on your arms.*

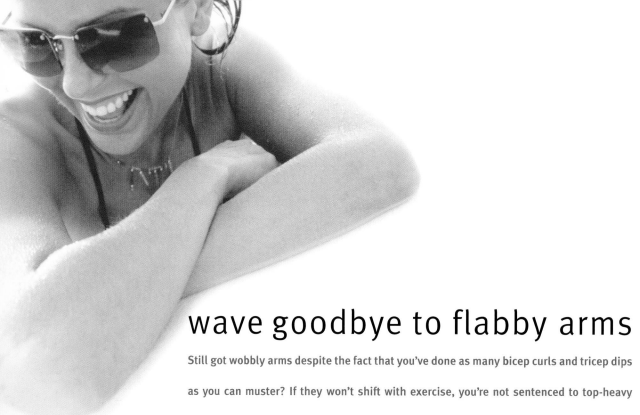

wave goodbye to flabby arms

Still got wobbly arms despite the fact that you've done as many bicep curls and tricep dips as you can muster? If they won't shift with exercise, you're not sentenced to top-heavy arms forever – there are some surgical options, too.

DITCH YOUR WINGS

There's nothing worse than waving to someone across the street and then noticing that your upper arm keeps on moving long after your hand has stopped waving. Okay, so this might be a little bit of an exaggeration, but that's certainly how it feels sometimes. For many women, being uncomfortable with this area of the body is particularly annoying in sunny weather, when all around are slipping into tanks and sleeveless tee-shirts. It's unclear why some women have flabby arms and others don't – obviously exercise has a lot to do with it, but many believe that so does genetics.

For a permanent solution to this arm-loathing problem, there are a couple of surgery options. Arm procedures are less talked about than other forms of surgery and the results are usually less dramatic than those you can expect to see elsewhere. Essentially the choice is between lipoplasty (or liposuction) to remove fat, or an 'arm lift' (brachioplasty) to get rid of excess skin. Both have their advantages and disadvantages.

So if arm surgery is so complicated, then why not just exercise? It's an important question, and one that should be answered only by first making the caveat that while surgery can be effective at reducing fat, it will never give your arms the tone and definition that's so attractive when peeping out of sleeveless shirts. Only exercise will do this. That said, if your saggy arms are the result of ageing skin, or major weight loss, exercise can improve but not eliminate the problem. Plus the older you are, arguably the longer it's going to take for you to see results from a regular arm workout.

ARM LIFTS

For most women – especially those who don't have masses of weight to lose – the arm lift (brachioplasty) is the best option. It tightens loose skin, and by stretching it, 'irons out' any rough or crêpey patches. It can be done under either local or general anaesthetic, and bruising and swelling normally last for no more than a couple of weeks, although you will have to wear a bandage or special compression garment for several weeks. You can exercise again after six weeks. For those women who think skin tightening is not quite enough but don't need to lose enough fat to warrant a full-blown lipoplasty procedure, small amounts of fat can sometimes be removed at the same time.

Brachioplasty's biggest disadvantage is its scar – it's usually a long, heavy, crooked line from the elbow to the armpit. Although it's on the underside of the arm, many women see the choice between flabby arms and unsightly scar as a difficult trade-off. Also, brachioplasty is not suitable for patients who have had a mastectomy (the arm's lymph drainage system may already be damaged) or those who suffer from excess sweat formation.

FIGHT THE FLAB

Where arms are disproportionately flabby, or where the patient is more than around 30 lbs (14 kilos) overweight, lipoplasty will give better results – although if the amount of skin you can pinch under the biceps is 5 cm (2 inches),

then there will still be flabby skin even after lipoplasty. An incision is made around the elbow and skin suctioned out in exactly the same way as in other parts of the body. You'll have bruising and swelling for about three weeks, after which your operation will have 'settled' and you'll be able to see your new shape – although it can often take a couple more months before you get the optimum results.

Many women worry that if they have fat removed from their arms, it will result in unsightly, flabby skin afterwards. Unless a large amount of fat has been removed, the skin tends to shrink back to fit its new size and will not sag – although you may be more prone to sagging in the years to come than you may otherwise have been. Advocates of the new ultrasound-enhanced lipoplasty claim that this is even better at helping skin to shrink, although the jury is still out on this.

Small-volume lipoplasty, sometimes referred to as liposculpture, is a relatively new development in arm surgery, and bridges the gap between brachioplasty and lipoplasty. Small incisions (around 3 mm/$\frac{1}{8}$ inch) are made at the elbow and other strategic points, depending on the areas being targeted. Pockets of fat where the arm meets the chest – front and back – are most frequently worked on, but other areas such as the wrists and elbows are also candidates. Only small amounts of fat are removed, using a very fine cannula or syringe.

Small-volume lipoplasty is excellent for 'finishing off' a job of 'regular' lipoplasty or for sorting out minor niggles – but as with its larger-volume counterpart, it can be expensive, complicated and painful. Your arms would have to really upset you for you to consider SVL on its own.

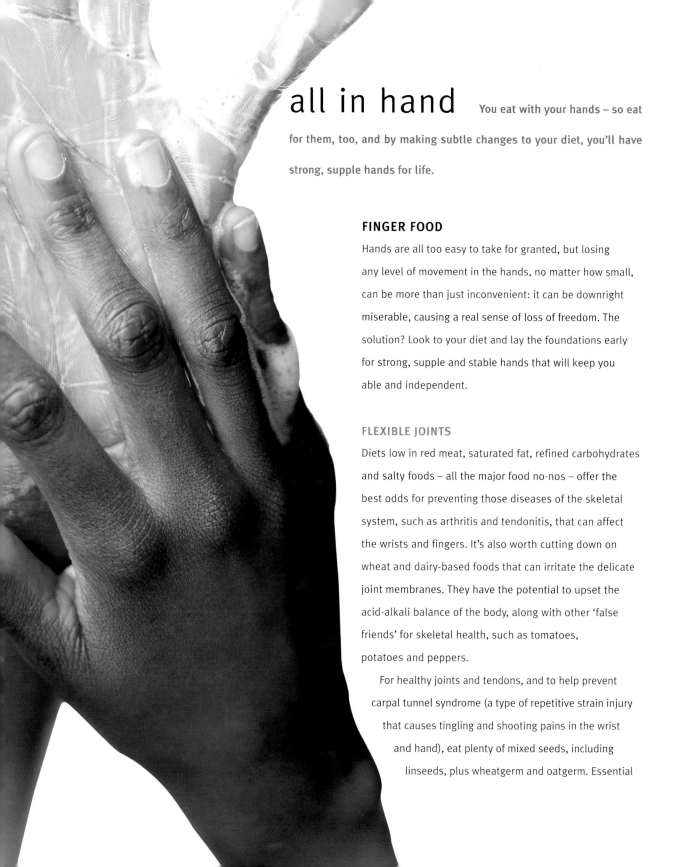

all in hand

You eat with your hands – so eat for them, too, and by making subtle changes to your diet, you'll have strong, supple hands for life.

FINGER FOOD

Hands are all too easy to take for granted, but losing any level of movement in the hands, no matter how small, can be more than just inconvenient: it can be downright miserable, causing a real sense of loss of freedom. The solution? Look to your diet and lay the foundations early for strong, supple and stable hands that will keep you able and independent.

FLEXIBLE JOINTS

Diets low in red meat, saturated fat, refined carbohydrates and salty foods – all the major food no-nos – offer the best odds for preventing those diseases of the skeletal system, such as arthritis and tendonitis, that can affect the wrists and fingers. It's also worth cutting down on wheat and dairy-based foods that can irritate the delicate joint membranes. They have the potential to upset the acid-alkali balance of the body, along with other 'false friends' for skeletal health, such as tomatoes, potatoes and peppers.

For healthy joints and tendons, and to help prevent carpal tunnel syndrome (a type of repetitive strain injury that causes tingling and shooting pains in the wrist and hand), eat plenty of mixed seeds, including linseeds, plus wheatgerm and oatgerm. Essential fatty acids in oily fish are, of course, excellent for joints. Finally, remember that joints and nails alike aren't at their happiest if you're following a low-fat diet that doesn't contain enough essential fatty acids.

NAIL FOOD

Nails thrive on a constant supply of nutrients delivered by a good blood supply. Acute periods of illness, where circulation has been affected, show up on nails in the form of bumps, grooves and streaks. Put your circulation to the test by plunging hands into cold water (about 12°C/55°F) and leaving them there for twenty seconds, then seeing how long it takes them to warm up. Fingers that are still white after ten minutes may indicate a circulation problem. White or dull-looking nails are obvious signs of poor circulation – healthy nails should look pink. If your nails look very dark brown, this is also cause for concern and you should have them checked by a doctor. Some medications may cause nail discolouration. In addition, a melanoma (the most serious type of skin cancer) could be growing on the nail bed, making the nail itself look brown. Yellow-tinged nails may be caused by nail polish staining, nicotine staining from smoking, or by general dehydration. Weak nails may signify anaemia or liver problems, and again, if you're worried, you should show them to your doctor.

In the same way that optimum levels of nutrients can strengthen nails, consuming too few of the right vitamins and minerals can put nail beds at risk from disease, letting fungal and other infections follow and leaving nails marked, ridged, yellow-tinged or misshaped. If your nail problems are more to do with dry, brittle nails and general flakiness, they're most likely to be caused by daily wear and tear than by nutrient deficiency.

The biggest myth surrounding nail health is that calcium helps to strengthen nails. It doesn't. This mistaken belief is thought to stem from the fact that calcium is so good for bones and teeth. That part is undoubtedly true – but the fact that nails themselves contain such minute quantities of calcium goes some way towards explaining why research has detected no discernible effect on the nails when calcium intake is stepped up.

The misguided championing of calcium as a wonder-treatment for nails has kept the true star nail nutrient out of the limelight: zinc. Leukonychia (white spots on the nail) can occur due to a lack of zinc, and many women who experience soft nails during pregnancy are advised to increase their zinc intake. The good news is that the levels needed, though significant, are small, and can easily be provided through regular helpings of red meat, shellfish and eggs. Zinc also helps the body to process essential fatty acids, which also help keep nails at the optimum levels of moisturisation. Women who take evening primrose oil often notice an improvement in their nails.

Though less significant, iron and selenium can also benefit the strength and appearance of the nails. Iron is useful when nails are brittle, and selenium will help problems with ridged nails. Ridges occur most often when stress or illness has caused nails to stop growing, then start again later, although they can also be a sign of a fungal infection. There's also anecdotal evidence that weak-nail sufferers have found ginkgo biloba to be of help.

beautiful hands: nailing the problem

Luxurious hand creams and pretty nail polishes may keep your hands looking gorgeous, but only you can keep them strong. Finger fitness might sound like the last word in exercise madness, but when it comes to supple, healthy and young-looking hands, these easy exercises can really help.

HANDY FOR WORK...

If you're interested in hand and finger exercises as a way to help with or compensate for large amounts of typing that you do for your job, it's worth taking a look at your working posture first. If you're slouching, twisting or unbalanced as you type, you're likely to be stopping your back, shoulder and upper arm muscles from working properly, forcing your hands and forearms to work harder than they need to.

Once you're sitting up straight, with your feet flat to the floor, your elbows close in and your keyboard straight in front of you, then you can begin to think about your hands. Keep hands slightly arched like little spiders, and don't let your wrists rest on your desk – it will force the fingers to take even more of the strain (if you're prone to this, look out for specially designed foam wrist-rests, which can help).

These handy tips can all help you avoid carpal tunnel syndrome, the repetitive strain injury common to typists and those who work for long periods with a mouse, pen or calculator. This debilitating condition occurs when the tendons in the wrist compress the nerve that runs through the 'tunnel' from wrist to hand. Exercises, though, will further strengthen your fingers and render them able to withstand all that hard work. Each hand contains thirty-four muscles – so it's worth giving them a workout from time to time.

A good exercise for finger strengthening, which feels good when performed a few times during breaks from typing, is this: touch your left and right hand fingers and thumbs together, then stretch and flex your typing fingers, first bringing them close together, then stretching them far apart. You can repeat as quickly as you like, and after about twenty repetitions, your fingers should feel revitalised and more agile.

ALWAYS HANDY...

Even if typing isn't a major part of your job, you'll certainly benefit from hand exercises. They increase circulation to those often hard-to-reach extremities, keeping tissues and tendons well nourished, staving off illness and helping to heal cuts and bruises that so often appear on hard-working hands. It may also even be possible to ensure that your fingers actually look leaner, too – so you can show them off with fab rings and nail polishes.

Finger exercises can also ensure a tighter grip – useful for things like bike riding or tennis – and also a firmer, stronger one good for unscrewing stubborn lids and screwing them back on again. In short, you'd be lost without full use of your flexible, versatile hands, so it pays to keep them trim. Handy, you might say!

HAND EXERCISES

To maintain flexible hands, try these exercises anytime, anywhere. They can be done easily at your desk — ideal if you work on a keyboard for long periods of time.

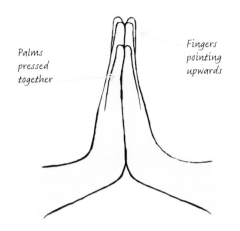

Palms pressed together

Fingers pointing upwards

1. Wrist mobility

The wrist is the vital starting point for good hand flexibility. As we age, it's particularly susceptible to softening and even breaking. In yoga, the 'prayer' position, a 'resting' pose that you return to time and again, is excellent for strengthening the wrist.

As the name suggests, it simply involves standing up straight, palms pressed together with fingertips pointing upwards. Do not let your hands lean into your chest; instead, feel the natural balance of your arms as the weight of your hands is evenly distributed between your wrists.

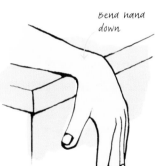

Bend hand down

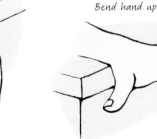

Bend hand up

2. Wrist mobility

Rest your elbow and forearm on a table, but make sure your hand is hanging

easily over the edge. Without moving your arm, simply bend your hand down, fingertips pointing to the floor, then up, fingertips pointing to the ceiling. **REPEAT** ten times.

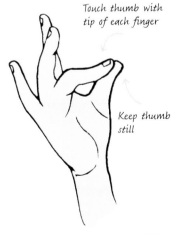

Touch thumb with tip of each finger

Keep thumb still

3. Fingers

Simply making a tight fist, holding it for a few seconds, then releasing will warm hands, stimulate circulation and prepare them for exercise. (Keep nails fairly short for this or they will dig in to your palms.)

Next, take each finger in turn and bend it three times: once at the tip, then in the middle, then at the base, stretching it forward so that it touches as near as possible the middle of the palm. Then do the whole thing in reverse.

4. Fingers

Finally, to keep your fingers really agile, take your thumb and, keeping it still, let each finger tip touch the tip of your thumb in turn. Repeat several times on each hand and, for variety, do the exercise on both hands together.

helping hands

The skin on your hands ages ten times faster than the skin on your face – and you thought your face caused you problems. Though there are thousands of products designed to help your face, hand preparations and their myriad ingredients are less well known. Here's what you need to know.

GOT TIME ON YOUR HANDS?

First things first: when it comes to looking after your hands and protecting them against the ravages of time, we're principally talking about the backs of your hands. The skin on your palms is different to skin elsewhere on your body: it has no hairs, for a start, and is much tougher considering its supreme levels of sensitivity. Palms sweat, so it's vital not to use an occlusive (pore-clogging) moisturiser (no petroleum jelly-based products) and don't worry about exfoliating – save that for the backs of the hands.

TREATMENT CREAMS

Most of the problems associated with hand ageing are the same ones we're used to dealing with on our faces: dehydration first, followed by cumulative exposure damage – as caused by UVA rays in sunlight. The bad news is that UVA rays can even penetrate glass, so there's no escape even if you're sitting by a window or driving.

The sun does more than just cause wrinkles, though – it's also responsible for those dark spots (sometimes called 'liver spots', 'sun spots' or 'age spots', but their real name is 'lentigines') that sometimes appear on the backs of the hands. They're harmless – just unsightly – unless they are changing colour or getting bigger or thickening, when it's worth getting them checked out.

For milder spots, there are treatment creams available, most of which involve skin-peeling agents, such as alpha hydroxy acids (AHAs), beta hydroxy acids, Retin-A or vitamin K. In their purest forms, they need to be treated as medication and applied once a day for around six months. AHA peels are a stronger alternative, working just like facial peels, as is liquid nitrogen therapy, where marks are spot frozen and the pigmented cells destroyed.

For prevention, it's the same as your face, an SPF15 cream should be fine and you don't need to wear it every day if you don't feel it's essential. You can now get some good purpose-designed hand creams that have SPFs and anti-dark spot complexes in them – they're lovely, but remember that the regular sun protection cream that you slap all over your body will work just as well against wrinkles.

ON THE NAIL

Nail disorders can take many forms: swelling, darkening, lightening, lifting from the nail bed, ridges, dents, spots and flaking. Unhygienic salon equipment or false nails are major culprits, but you can also catch nail disorders if you're constantly subjecting your hands to water. Many are difficult to treat – but with patience, topical anti-bacterial or anti-fungal applications can clear them up. These work by creating a watertight seal over the infected areas to cut off

Structure of nail and finger tip

Nail folds – the folds of the skin that frame and support the nail on three sides.

Nail plate – the visible part of the nail.

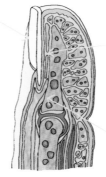

Nail bed – the skin beneath the nail plate.

Cuticle – tissue that overlaps the plate and rims the base of the nail.

Lunula – part of the matrix – the whitish, half-moon shape at the base of the nail, usually most pronounced on the thumb.

Matrix – the area under the cuticle, the hidden part of the nail unit where growth takes place.

NAILS are a good indicator of your general health. Look out for abnormalities such as discolouration or separation of the nail from its bed.

their oxygen supply. Both the skin surrounding the nails and the delicate skin of the nail bed can become infected by bacteria or fungi. Paronychia refers to an infection of the skin around the nails, often caused by a torn hangnail. Red, swollen and painful skin around the margins of the nail are a sign of possible infection. Relief may be obtained by soaking the fingertip in warm water several times a day. If the redness and swelling persist or if there is any sign of pus, have a doctor look at it.

Onychia is an infection of the nail bed itself, and it often results in loss of the nail. These infections require a doctor's attention because the area is covered by the nail plate. It's difficult to get medication to it, and the waterproof covering provided by the nail plate makes a fertile environment for the growth of bacteria and fungi. Women who wear artificial nails are particularly prone to onychia.

If you feel pain or pressure under a nail or an area of your nail takes on a dark greenish tinge, show it to your doctor. Other signs that should send you to the doctor are discolouration and lifting of the nail plate. A doctor may prescribe soaks, a topical ointment or medication you take by mouth. He or she might remove the nail plate to make it easier to treat the area. The nail will grow back in time.

Preventative measures are best. Always remove all soap from your nails, and dry them properly. Don't keep your nails submerged for too long, and avoid direct contact with strong detergents – use rubber gloves. Nail biting is also out – not only does it look messy, it makes it easy for bacteria to spread from your fingers to your mouth and back again. Also, remember that beauticians and salon nail technicians aren't qualified to deal with nail infections – your doctor should be your first port of call.

THE PERFECT MANICURE

When it comes to looking super-groomed, well-kept hands and nails are the ultimate finishing touch. Here's the fuss-free way to make your hands your best accessory.

SMOOTH

Soft hands create the right impression – they signify kindness, gentleness and warmth. Keep yours soft by exfoliating once a week – it needn't be a step too far on your ever-growing list of beauty chores, either. When you exfoliate your face (which you may be doing once a week anyway), just scoop a little extra product out and rub it over the tops and undersides of your hands. Sweeping away the dead skin cells will ease any rough patches and prime hands to drink up all the precious moisture that will follow when you apply hand cream (or any ultra-rich moisturiser – the kind you'd use on your feet, not your face). In fact, if your daily hand cream contains an SPF, it's worth using a richer, non-SPF cream at night to maximise the moisturising process. Some high-tech hand creams contain cell-loosening ingredients, for example AHAs. These are useful for older hands, but don't reapply as frequently as a non-'peeling' one. For a once-a-week treat, to compete with the super-hydrating paraffin wax offered by salons with a warm oil wrap: warm olive oil to slightly above room temperature, massage it into hands and then wrap in plastic film.

SHAPED

When applying hand cream, don't miss out your nails – nails are actually layers of modified skin cells and they benefit just as much from an extra moisture boost to compensate for all the abuse they get in the name of general wear and tear. Spend a minute massaging your lotion right into each cuticle, too – cuticle dryness is the major cause of hangnails. Next, shape your cuticles – it will reduce dryness and make nails look longer, too. You can buy special AHA cuticle creams for the purpose, which prevent cuticles from becoming too thick. Resist the temptation to cut them – you'll risk exposing your nail beds to infection. If they're ragged or long, gently push them back with a warm wet flannel – manicurists use a round-edged tool called an orange stick and these are available in chemists and beauty salons. Push cuticles back tentatively, bit by bit, using small circular movements to sweep away any residue. Only now can you get out the nail or cuticle clippers and trim any hangnails.

SMART

The shape you file your nails into comes down to individual choice: some people like the fashionable statement of square-ended nails; others like the natural appearance of rounded tips. Most people go for something in-between, dubbed the 'squoval', which not only makes nails look groomed and tidy, but is also fairly easy to achieve. Simply trim the nails to the desired length (the shorter you keep them, the stronger they will be) and then with a nail file, work at each corner to take the 'edges' off. Despite varying prices, nail files are all very similar – best to buy cheaper and replace frequently for maximum precision. Always file from the side of the nail towards the centre, never forwards and backwards – you'll weaken the nail if you do this. Next, time for the fun part – nail polish. Every time you open a bottle of nail polish, you're exposing it to evaporation, which causes the formulation to thicken. Most polishes are past their best after around six months, although it is possible to prolong their life slightly by thinning them down with a few drops of nail polish remover. It's a good idea to apply a clear base coat before your colour – it creates a smooth, glassy surface for application and, with dark colours, stops the colour staining your nails. After two coats of your chosen colour, add another clear layer to keep your polish chip-free.

STYLISH

False nails have come a long way since the days when fake white, super-thick pieces of plastic were the only option. These days, there's really no way of knowing – especially with the latest false nails, which are made of mouldable synthetics and are 'painted' on to your existing nails so there's no chance of a giveaway join. After two weeks, you'll need to go back to the salon for a 'filler' – to paint in the gaps where nail growth has occurred – but other than that, maintenance is minimal. Less high-tech but equally durable are regular acrylic nails, where separate pieces are applied and then quickly 'baked' on by placing each finger under an ultraviolet light. The same sort of up-keep is required. And if you find the time and expense of salon nails daunting, don't dismiss at-home varieties – road-tested by nail addicts and able to last three or four days at a time comfortably. Now your only dilemma is which colour to paint them....

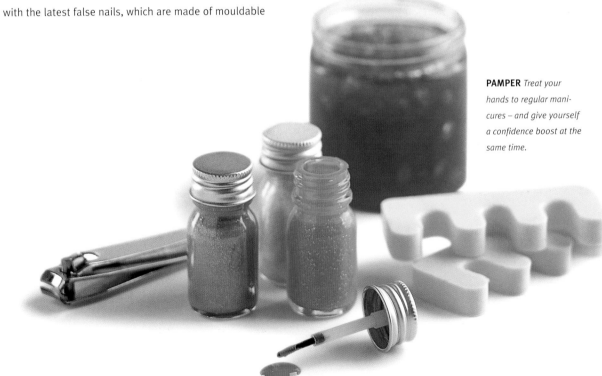

PAMPER *Treat your hands to regular mani-cures – and give yourself a confidence boost at the same time.*

hand surgery

When your hands start to look older than your face, it could be time to consider hand surgery. So just what can medical procedures do for your hands – is it safe and what kind of results can you expect? Arm yourself with the facts you need to help your hands.

COSMETIC PROCEDURES

Until very recently, hand surgery was almost always performed out of necessity – for joint disorders, for example, or the nerve entrapped by carpal tunnel syndrome. Now, having all but sorted out their faces, women – and their surgeons – are looking for procedures that will sort out aesthetic concerns, too.

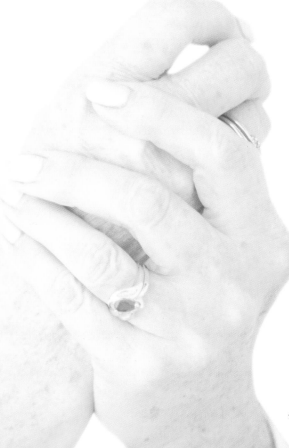

GIVE YOUR HANDS A BOOST

When hands age, the tissue beneath the surface becomes thinner and less springy. The overlying skin, which used to cover a larger surface area, therefore becomes wrinkled and saggy. Boosting the hands' depleted tissue will not only make them look healthier, but will iron out some of those wrinkles, too. 'Filler' injections, which are now commonly used on the face to 'plump up' the skin and soften the appearance of wrinkles, have therefore found their way down to the hands.

Whereas facial injections are most often performed with collagen, hand injections are most frequently carried out with fat cells taken from other parts of your body (known as autologous fat injections) – they're thought to last longer than most synthetic substances. Using your own fat means you avoid the potential of allergic reaction sometimes seen with collagen. With injected fat, the surgeon is able to shape and 'sculpt' the area to get the desired contour.

It depends on the size and position of the area treated, but using your own fat can last for anywhere between one and five years.

HOLDING BACK THE YEARS *Older hands can be enhanced with surgery – filler injections and chemical peels are just some of the treatments now on offer.*

As you'd expect, very little fat is actually needed from the 'donor' site – surgeons usually take between 20 and 50 cc of fat in a 'small-volume lipoplasty' operation that's done with a syringe – but only half of the harvested amount will, once cleaned and refined, end up being used. Five or six tiny incisions are made at the wrist and around the back of the hand for the needles to go through, and the injected fat then weaves its way round the tissue and veins. The whole operation can be performed under local anaesthetic. Hands are, however, notoriously complicated structures, so it's important to find a well-practised surgeon. Irregular deposits of fat – leading to strange bulges – are not impossible, nor is misjudging the quantities of fat needed, meaning you could end up with too little, or worse, too much.

Happily, fat injections can also help make veins less prominent. However, if raised, blueish veins are your biggest concern, your surgeon may suggest sclerotherapy, a procedure that has been used for years in the treatment of spider veins on the legs. A tiny needle is used to inject a saline 'sclerosing' solution into the vein. This salt-water solution irritates the veins, causing them to shrink back from the surface so that they're no longer as visible. You'll normally need multiple injections along the length of the vein, but it's a fairly fast procedure (usually less than an hour) requiring just local anaesthetic.

In the case of leg veins, particularly smaller, 'spider' ones, however, another type of treatment has all but taken over: laser therapy. Laser treatments have the advantage of being fast, precise and, of course, non-invasive. Used for hands, you may need several treatments (with a gap of a few weeks in between), but can expect near-total elimination. The effects may not last forever, but can remain for up to around ten years.

REJUVENATION THERAPY

Lasers are also being increasingly used on the hands because they have so many all-round benefits. They are very good at eliminating dark brown 'age spots' – one of the biggest concerns for women with ageing hands, and a phenomenon that until now has never been very easy to treat. Traditional bleaching methods seldom had much success at lightening pigmentation caused by ageing and excess sun exposure, but for many women, laser surgery can seem an extreme (and expensive) solution to the problem.

Chemical peels, so popular now for the face, are also very useful for rejuvenating the appearance of the hands. A mild peel can lighten dark spots and also help resurface the backs of the hands to eliminate dry-looking, crêpey skin. A medium or deep chemical peel will have a more profound effect on age spots, especially when mixed with a bleaching agent – also now a possibility. One word of warning though – for such a small area and such tried-and-tested treatments, recovering from any kind of hand surgery can be surprisingly lengthy. As one of our primary methods of touch, it's no surprise that our hands are highly sensitive, meaning post-operative pain is, for some people, a big issue. With all of these procedures, hands will be taped up for several days and sensitive for up to a month. Before you make any decisions, discuss the options with a surgeon, who'll be able to tell you how deep your lines or pigmentation are – this could impact the treatment you choose.

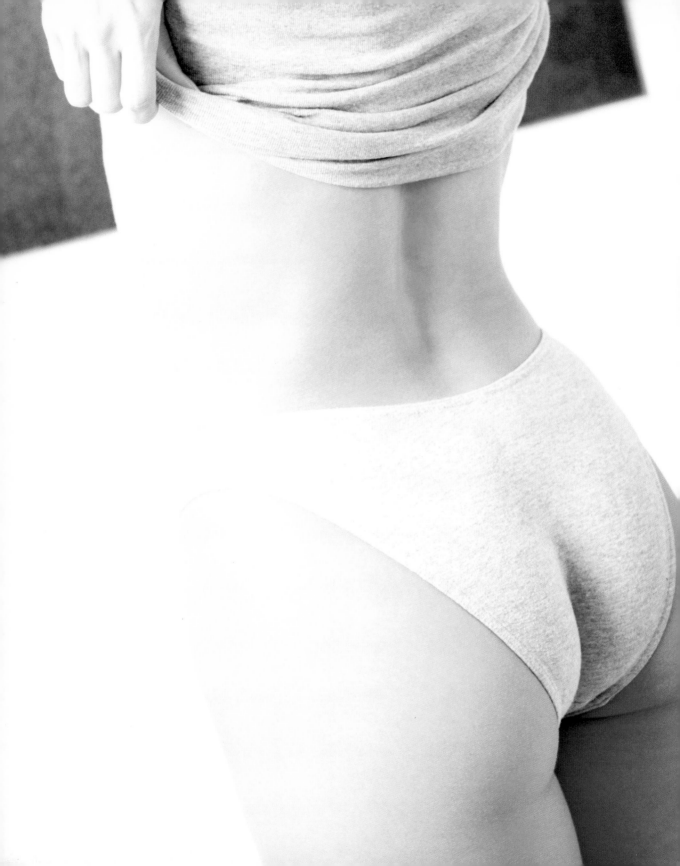

bottom

When we're thinking about our bodies, sooner or later we always end up lamenting our bottoms. Too big, too small, too flat, too round, too lumpy, out of shape...the list is endless. So what's the solution? Is it possible to spot-treat your behind with exercise and a special butt-busting diet? This section continues the theme that you'll get the most from your body when you think of it as a whole. That's why each specially targeted heading, whether it's looking at trimming hips, toning thighs or even revitalising put-upon feet, will take you through the key physical factors to bear in mind for long-term improvement to your lower half, such as leg-stretching exercises that will give the appearance of longer limbs or diet tips to banish water retention. And then there are quick-fix treatments, such as the perfect pedicure or cellulite wrap, that will spur you on along the way.

dieting for hips and thighs When it comes to weight loss,

why are hips so stubborn, with so many of us suffering from the much-lamented 'pear' shape? Can eating the right food really help? What, if anything, will specifically shift the weight from our hips? Read on for the answers, and discover why an ample bottom may not be as bad for you as you think.

HOW FAT ACCUMULATES

The fact that so many of us bemoan the heaviness of our bottoms and thighs is no surprise: for women, heavy hips and thighs are normal – a svelte lower half is the exception, not the rule. The classic 'pear' shape is a typically female phenomenon because oestrogen, the hormone that women have in abundance until menopause, encourage us to store excess fat on our hips, thighs and bottoms. After the menopause, when oestrogen levels dip, it's common for fat to accumulate on the waist instead of the hips – more like it does in men.

The discovery of several 'fat' genes has recently led experts to suspect that certain aspects of weight gain may be genetically predetermined, so you might be right in thinking that you've inherited one or both of your parents' tendencies for a big bottom. That said, the genetic link is most apparent when it comes to general, all-over weight gain as opposed to specific areas, and it is more commonly noted in obesity: a child with two obese parents has an 80 per cent chance of growing up obese. For the lower degrees of excess weight that plague most of us, though, our own calorie intake versus energy expenditure, not our genetic make-up, is thought to be the overriding factor in how much weight we amass.

BOTTOM HEAVY

So now we know what the weight on our hips and thighs is doing there, the question is what can we do about it? Just as the hips and thighs are often the first area that extra weight gravitates towards, it's also often the case that this is the hardest area of the body to shift weight away from. Roughly speaking, women lose weight from top to bottom – so you'll usually see it coming off your face, bust, then stomach before it finally leaves your hips and thighs. This means that if you are a 'pear' shape, that even when you do lose weight, you'll often find you're simply a thinner 'pear' than you were before.

Then, horror of horrors, there's the fact that the thinner you are, the harder it is to shift those last few pounds. In general, if you weigh 16 stones (100 kilos) you can safely and easily lose 4 lbs (1.8 kilos) a week, but if you're 10 stones (64 kilos), 1 lb a week – at most – should be your aim. At this point it's time to start stepping up – literally – your exercise routine to try and tighten up your thighs and bottom. The bottom line is this: no one's going to lose weight from their hips and thighs overnight.

So where do these countless diets that profess to spot-treat the stubborn hip and thigh area come into the equation? It's worth remembering two things about them.

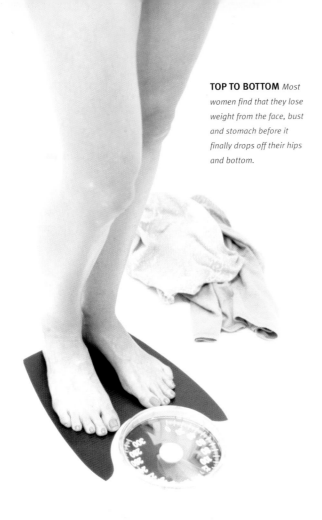

TOP TO BOTTOM *Most women find that they lose weight from the face, bust and stomach before it finally drops off their hips and bottom.*

shift weight from your hips, a low-fat diet will – but of course you'll lose the weight all over, not just from your hips. If it doesn't get its fat supply through food, your body will produce an enzyme called lipoprotein lipase, which increases fat storage in your body – so when you do eat some fat, it could hang around longer than it would otherwise have done. For sensible weight loss, try and keep your daily fat intake between 10 and 30 per cent of your total calorific intake. But before all this talk of 'inevitable' fat storage on the hips starts to make you too gloomy, consider this: having a big bottom might not be quite the burden you think it is. A study looking at the hip sizes of around 1,400 women found that those whose excess weight settles on their hips and bottom were less likely to suffer from diabetes and heart disease than those whose extra weight is distributed more evenly around the body. It should be pointed out that all the women tested were of average weight to begin with – there's an obvious link between very large hips and heart disease.

If you have a particularly sedentary lifestyle – taking the bus to work every day, doing a job that involves sitting down all day long, and then getting back on the bus to come home and sit in front of a television – it's inevitable that your bottom will become a little heavy. At work, try to make sure that you get out of your seat at least once every hour: if you work at a computer, then your eyes and back muscles will benefit as well. When you are sitting at your desk, try to keep your feet raised above the ground slightly. You can get special footrests for this purpose, or you can use piles of old magazines (they'll give you something to read at lunchtime as well!).

Number one: no diet can spot-treat particular areas of the body – the only thing that can do that is lipoplasty. Number two: most of these diets will still produce overall weight loss (when followed correctly), which will eventually get round to the hips and thighs. It's up to you whether you see this extra weight loss as a bonus or a swindle.

Most of the 'hip and thigh' diets are low-fat, high-carb and are coupled with a stringent exercise regime (which is the thing that makes the difference to your bottom, hips and thighs specifically). It's true that if anything will help

the dimples you don't want

As many as 90 per cent of women could be affected by cellulite to some degree. The trick to treating it? Know your enemy. That means cutting through the vast numbers of conflicting opinions until you get to the bottom of the matter. Food, water, toxins and exercise all have a part to play. Here's what you need to know.

CELLULITE – FACT OR FICTION?

We've all heard the cries from medical experts: cellulite doesn't exist. Okay, so the lumpy, dimpled areas on our bottoms are just figments of our imagination – skimpy bikinis here we come. Not convinced? Don't worry – now that we know more about the causes of cellulite, it's not only being recognised by more members of the medical profession, we're also closer than ever to knowing how best to combat it.

THE TRUTH ABOUT CELLULITE

Cellulite has nothing to do with being overweight – although it may look worse when there's more fat underneath the skin's surface. It also cuts through age barriers (though older women may be more susceptible as they lose skin elasticity, giving the cellulite more room to manoeuvre). Very few men get cellulite because their connective tissue is tough because of their testosterone levels, and their excess weight doesn't settle on their hips and thighs.

So what's going on? The story begins with the fat cells in your buttocks and thighs. They lie just below the skin and have the capacity to store huge amounts of fat (about half of your body's total fat is kept here). When you're young, they are neatly lined up in rows beneath the dermal layer of your skin, each one housed in its own little chamber.

As we age, fluctuating hormones can cause the fat cells to expand. Of course, weight gain is also responsible for this – but cellulite is thought to develop primarily during periods of hormonal change, such as puberty, pregnancy, menopause and even the first few months of taking birth control pills. The vertical strands of collagen that hold the little chambers of fat and surrounding tissues together are tough and rigid, and won't bend to accommodate the expanding fat, so the fat pockets bulge and 'spill' through the tissue, causing lumps to appear. So, the fat that forms cellulite is really no different from the fat found anywhere else on the body.

Another factor is the circulation, although the extent of its involvement is hotly debated. Some experts say that toxin build-up is a major contributor to cellulite, and that if your circulation is sluggish, blood and lymphatic vessels can leak into the surrounding tissue, causing swelling and preventing nutrients reaching the fatty tissue so that toxins cannot be drained away so easily. Broken, weak or varicose veins can hinder good drainage, as can a poor lymph system and stress. You can drink lots of water to combat this.

Others argue that if toxins play such a big part in cellulite, it would also be prevalent in men. They argue that drinking excessive quantities of water will only encourage

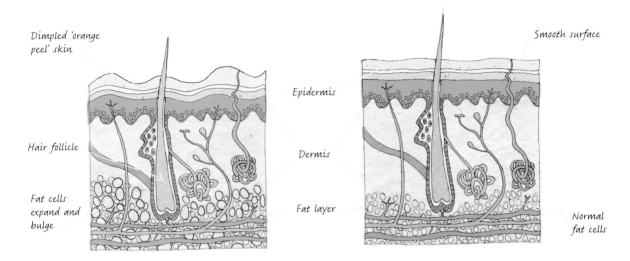

Dimpled 'orange peel' skin

Hair follicle

Fat cells expand and bulge

Epidermis

Dermis

Fat layer

Smooth surface

Normal fat cells

Cellulite

Normal skin

Structure of cellulite

cellulite – it's proven that cellulite contains high numbers of proteoglycans (molecules that attract water) and has higher levels of water than other fat cells in the body. Whatever your conclusion, it's fair to say that the classic ingredients of a healthy diet – 2 litres ($4\frac{1}{4}$ pints) of water a day, fresh fruit and vegetables, and avoiding too much alcohol and spicy food – coupled with circulation-boosting exercise – is best. That way you'll be giving your body every chance of shifting every kind of fat on its own.

CONQUERING CELLULITE

If you don't buy the 'toxins build-up' theory, then logically you won't have any time for the 'anti-cellulite' tablets that claim to help with drainage and circulation. You're right to be sceptical: there are currently no guidelines governing cellulite products. If you do want to try them, make sure you

choose an all-natural variety – it will probably contain circulation-boosting ingredients like ginkgo biloba, horse chestnut and grape seed extract – and don't pay over the odds. It's almost certainly better to add cellulite-shifters – of which there are plenty – to your meals than to take supplements designed to rush everything through your system.

Onions, garlic, ginger and fennel are some of the best cellulite busters, as are aubergines, bananas, seafood, lentils, beans and peas. Unsurprisingly, unsaturated fats such as cold-pressed seed and vegetable oils, raw nuts and seeds are preferable to saturated fats (such as fatty meats), hydrogenated fats (processed oils that are not cold pressed) and trans-fatty acids (including smoked meats, preserved meats and dairy products). Eat fibre-rich foods like fruit, vegetables and cereals and cut down on salt – it can lead to water retention.

THIGH HOPES

Contrary to popular belief, the thighs can be trimmed dramatically (although normally only after most of the other body parts have been slimmed down). They're made up of four major thigh muscle groups: the hamstrings in the back of the thigh, which work to bend the knee; the adductors – the inner thigh muscles; the quadriceps at the front of the thigh, which help straighten the knee; and the hip flexors at the front of the pelvis, which help you raise your thighs.

TONE YOUR THIGHS

Thigh toning calls for a fairly tenacious, aggressive approach – but this doesn't have to mean hours of pumping iron and endless lunges. One of the good things – and there aren't many – about our thighs is that we use the thigh muscles in practically every physical activity. You can make a difference to your thighs before you hit the gym by simply incorporating a few extra elements into your daily routine.

Walking, in-line skating and cycling are good ways to start. Turn a cycle ride into a thigh-focused workout by leading with your heel as you pedal and strapping your feet onto the pedals using toe clips. Without them, you'll primarily be engaging only the quadriceps, but with toe clips your hamstrings will get a workout, too.

Swimming is a useful thigh trimmer. Front crawl, not the gentler action of breaststroke, will provide the most powerful exercise, but don't think it's all about kicking your legs in a fast and furious manner. Long, fluid kicks are better – and remember to kick out right from the hip, not just from the knees. That way your hips, thighs, bottom and even stomach will be involved in the workout. If you're a gym-class fan, try Tae Bo for weight shifting or kickboxing for toning.

MOVES TO TRY

After exercising your thighs, stretch the muscles so that they don't become too bulky.

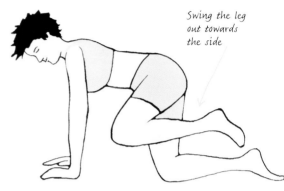

Swing the leg out towards the side

1. Leg extends

On all fours, lift one knee up towards the chest and then swing back, taking a straight line and extending the leg until its fully outstretched behind you. Either return the leg to its start position, knee on the ground, or increase the difficulty by then swinging the leg out to the side like a chicken wing and then returning the knee to the floor.

2. Wide step-outs

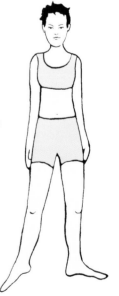

Effective when done straight after aerobic exercise. From a standing position, step out around 30 cm (12 inches) to the right with the right foot, then to the left with the left foot, to make a 'V' step. Quickly return the right foot, then the left foot, to the centre and repeat twenty times.

3. Leg lifts

Lie on your back with arms flat to the floor. Bend one leg, but make sure the foot is still flat to the floor. Raise the other leg until it is the same height as the bent knee, hold and lower. Repeat twenty times. Next, lie on your side with the leg that's on the floor slightly bent. Keeping the other leg straight, raise it 30 cm (12 inches), hold, then lower.

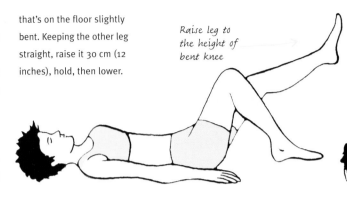

Raise leg to the height of bent knee

4. Curtsey lunges

Stand up straight, hands on hips. Take your right foot and step backwards diagonally behind your left leg. The knee of your right leg should be in line with the heel of the left foot. Tighten the gluteal muscles and as you do so, lower the right knee towards (but not touching) the ground. Hold, then return right leg to the centre and repeat for the left leg. **REPEAT** five times on each side.

Step back-wards behind left leg

Right knee should be in line with left heel

5. Hamstring stretch

Place your left foot one pace in front of the right. Link your hands and place them on your left thigh, letting it take your weight. Hold for fifteen seconds.

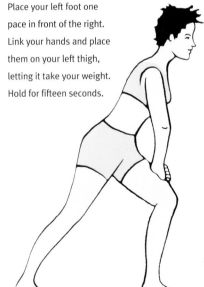

Press hips forward

6. Hip flexor stretch

Kneeling down, extend your right leg so its heel rests on the floor. Press hips forward so your left hip bears your weight. Hold for fifteen seconds, then change sides.

WORK THAT BUTT

These are the moves you need for a serious bottom workout. Remember to start with a warm-up – walk up a hill or on a treadmill set for an incline for at least ten minutes.

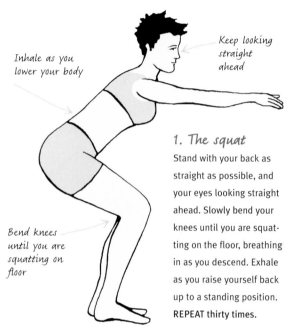

Inhale as you lower your body

Keep looking straight ahead

Bend knees until you are squatting on floor

1. The squat
Stand with your back as straight as possible, and your eyes looking straight ahead. Slowly bend your knees until you are squatting on the floor, breathing in as you descend. Exhale as you raise yourself back up to a standing position. **REPEAT thirty times.**

2. The lunge
Standing up straight, step your right foot a good stride's length in front of the left. Bend your knees, making sure that your right knee is in line with your right foot. The more weight you put on your right heel, the more work your glutes will be doing. **REPEAT twenty times.**

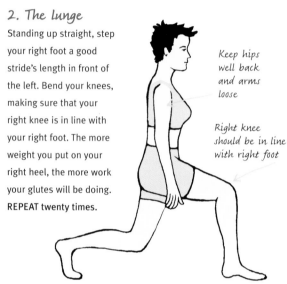

Keep hips well back and arms loose

Right knee should be in line with right foot

3. The plié squat
Stand up straight, hips back and abdominals tight, with feet more than shoulder width apart, toes turned out. Place your hands on your hips. Bend your knees and lower your body towards the floor. Knees should be in line with toes at all times, and as with lunges, you should push yourself back up from your heels. **REPEAT twenty times.**

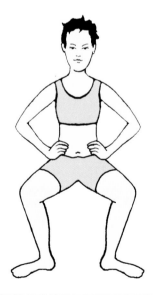

4. The butt lift
Lie on your back with your knees bent and your feet against a wall. With your arms flat, lift your bottom a few inches off the ground so that your legs are fully extended. Concentrate on pressing your heels into the wall and raising your hips another inch or so. Hold for a few moments, then release and gently lower your bottom back to the floor. **REPEAT fifteen times.**

5. The step-up

Another effective favourite. Use a bench, staircase, box or exercise step that will cause you to bend your knee at around 90 degrees when you step onto it. Standing at the foot of the bench, raise your right foot onto the bench and then bring the left one up to join it, exhaling as you do so. Now, return the right foot to the floor. The toning effect comes from controlling the descent as slowly as possible. Don't attempt step-ups if you suffer from knee pain. **REPEAT ten times on one leg, then the same with the other.**

6. The butt stretch

Sit on the floor, cross-legged, with your hands flat out behind you supporting your weight. Bring your left foot up onto your right knee and press down your left knee. Feel the stretch in your left buttock and hip. Hold for fifteen seconds, then swap sides.

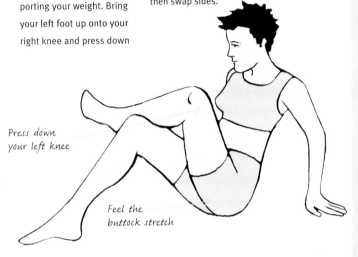

Press down your left knee

Feel the buttock stretch

7. Pilates leg, hips and buttock balancer

Lie on the floor, knees softly bent, feet flat to the floor. Breathe in, then out, pulling in your abs and raise your right knee but still bent at the knee. Your right calf is therefore raised but parallel to the floor. Breathe deeply, stretch your leg out so that it is straight, toes pointing upward. Breathe out, and flex your raised foot. Breathe in, and keeping your abs tight and back straight, lower the leg to the floor.

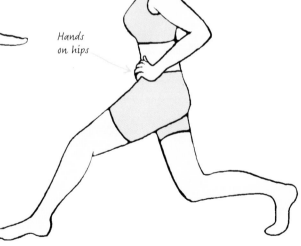

Support upper back with pillow

Shoulders back

Hands on hips

8. The yoga lunge

Stand up and step your right foot back as far as you can. Breathe deeply. Bring your hands down so that they are either side of your left foot, your upper body leaning forward. Place your right foot flat so that your weight is now resting on the upper side, not the ball of your foot. Bring the right foot alongside the left so that you are squatting down. Slowly return to standing position.

DO IT YOURSELF

Lumpy, wobbly or just unappealing hips and thighs? Lavish them with the attention of an easy self-massage – it can reward you with smoother skin and better circulation.

We know that we can't solve the problem of wobbly bits by massage alone; nor is it easy to set aside the time and money for regular massage treatments at beauty salons or day spas, even if they do leave you feeling like you're walking on air. Why not try a spot of self-massage? Working on your hips, thighs and parts of your buttocks is easy – and when combined with a healthy eating plan could make a real difference to your whole hip area. If you exercise regularly, this massage will also help those hard-working upper leg muscles.

WORK ON YOUR MUSCLES

A self hip and thigh massage can be as fast as a quick pummel as you get out of the bath or shower or as relaxing as a twenty-minute knead before bed. If you're planning to give yourself a massage last thing at night, have a bath instead of a shower to raise your body temperature, soften skin and really get your circulation pumping. Essential oils of eucalyptus, rosemary and orange will also help get toxins on the move. It's also a good idea to drink plenty of water – dehydrated muscles are less pliable and can also lead to stiffness after massage.

Begin by massaging your hamstrings, located at the back of your upper thighs. Sitting down on a hard surface (not your bed), bring your right leg up, foot still flat to the floor, and with your right hand, grasp the muscles underneath your right thigh and begin to jostle them gently from

side to side. Go right from the back of the knee to the crease where your thigh meets your bottom, then switch sides. For your quadriceps (front of the thighs), bend your leg again and with the heels of both palms, apply pressure to the muscles by pumping your hands up and down on your leg. For extra pressure, lean forward as you press in and again work from above the knee up to your hip area.

To massage your glutes (located in the hip area), you'll need to stand up. Working on both hips together, place your hands just below the flabbiest part of your hips and make circular movements around your hips, sweeping lightly on the 'downward' part of the circle and applying more pressure for the 'upward' movements. After circling for a few moments, lose the 'downward' moves and simply perform long, sweeping, upward strokes from the bottom of your hips up to the curve of your waist.

Next, simply move your hands round to your bottom and with one hand on each buttock, continue the upward sweeping strokes, applying as much pressure as is comfortable. As you get to the top of your buttocks, finish by bringing your hands out to the side of your buttocks as they finish the strokes – don't let them travel further up your back, where you might end up contorting your arms into an awkward position.

Finish off by lying down again – you can do this bit in bed if you like. You can gently massage your abdomen by lying flat on your back and using the fingertips of both hands to make small clockwise circles across your stomach and up to the base of your ribcage. Make sure it's at least a couple of hours since you ate your evening meal, though, and be sure not to press too hard at any point.

AND RELAX...

After your massage, if you're not going straight to bed, try resting in the yoga 'child pose'. It's a good way to give your body time to recover and – if you're doing it first thing in the morning – it also gives you a few moments to yourself before getting on with your day. Kneel down so that you are sitting on your heels, and slowly let your upper body roll forward so that it is parallel to the floor. Position your arms so that they are either stretching out straight in front of you, or so that they are behind you, running along the length of your curled-up body, palms facing up. This latter position is a good way to conserve your body heat.

Finally, for an energising boost that is particularly effective first thing in the morning, try a position that's taken from the principles of Ayurveda. Kneel on the floor, sitting on the back of your heels, hands on top of your thighs. As you inhale, tilt your hips and back forwards slightly, then rock gently backwards as you exhale. Repeat several times. This move aims to open your 'base chakra', which helps control your strength, endurance and energy supplies. The position might feel a little strange at first, but persevere with it: once you have tried it a few times, you will probably find that it is one of the most comfortable positions in which to relax. It also has the added advantage of keeping the weight off your over-burdened bottom.

TREAT YOURSELF *Diet and exercise are crucial in toning up the hips, thighs and bottom, but massage and gentle stretching will also help.*

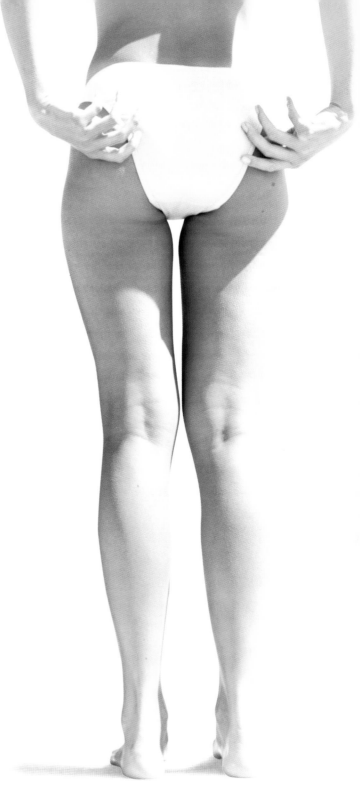

stand tall
Perfect legs are as much about attitude as appearance. Your legs may never be perfectly shapely and you may never achieve exquisitely shaped ankles, but give them the attention they deserve – in the form of a few simple exercises – and you can reap the benefits inside and out.

PERFECT PINS

When it comes to our legs, we can be pretty demanding about what we want. With bottoms it's usually just 'smaller' or 'rounder', with arms it's 'more definition' and with waists it's 'flatter', but for our legs we want just about everything going: toned and firm but not too bulky; shapely but not too wide and athletic; and strong but still graceful and elegant.

STRETCHING FOR SHAPELIER LEGS

While aerobic and resistance training are still the first port of call for building up muscle strength and definition (*see pages 150–51*), it's to stretches that fitness trainers are now turning in order to help their clients achieve the shapelier legs they've always wanted.

However, it's not as simple as saying that 'stretching elongates muscles where strength training compacts them, therefore for longer-looking legs, we must all do stretches'. The effect that stretches have on the joints is in increasing their range of movement, and that effect is pretty short-lived: it is generally believed to last somewhere between three and sixty minutes. What stretching can do is, over time, increase the muscles' capacity to be elongated before pain or damage set in, thereby making exercising safer and stiffness less likely.

In terms of making your legs look more shapely, though, stretching can have the important effect of 'normalising' the bulking effects of weight-bearing exercise. When you first begin exercising the legs, the muscles can appear to get bulkier very quickly – in a couple of weeks or so – though they'll 'tone down' later. In the meantime, this often puts people off.

That's not to say that resistance work can't also have the effect of elongating the leg muscles: hamstring exercises, for example, can help you achieve longer-looking legs and a slimmer bottom, and exercising your calves can give the appearance of shapelier ankles and knees.

Yoga is central to the new stretching craze and is particularly good for the legs. This is partly because of the yoga balances, which encourage strength, stamina and good posture. Tai chi is also excellent for balancing, although not specifically muscle toning. And a new fitness workout, the New York City Ballet Workout, is currently attracting the most attention from those wanting elegant dancer-style legs.

The NYC Ballet Workout involves stretching, strengthening exercises and a small amount of aerobic workout. It's based around ballet positions – ones that are particularly good for the legs include pliés (like open-legged squats) and arabesques (standing leg raises).

LEGS THAT FLY

Well-exercised legs should also have good circulation, which can be especially important when you're travelling. Deep vein thrombosis (DVT) can occur when the central blood vessels in the legs are compressed for extended periods, causing blood clots to develop.

Though DVT has been dubbed 'economy class syndrome', it has more to do with sitting still for hours at a time than with the width of your seat (although the backs of your legs are more likely to rest on the bottom of your chair where there's less leg room, which could be a contributing factor). Also, though no studies are as yet completed, it's thought that dehydration and the pressurised air in aircraft cabins also contribute to DVT.

Those most at risk from DVT include people who have recently had surgery, who suffer from blood disorders that can increase clotting, and women who are pregnant or taking the contraceptive pill. Smokers and those over the age of forty also have a slightly increased risk. Experts don't agree on what length of flight, if any, constitutes a risk from blood clots. Simple ways to minimise your risks: wear loose clothing, eat only small meals and drink plenty of water.

LEG EXERCISES

Don't cross your legs while seated, adjust your seat position every half an hour, and try and get up and move around every hour or so. Also, try these circulation-pumping in-seat exercises:

1. Foot pumps
Lift the knee towards the chest, then straighten it to its full range. **REPEAT several times then swap legs.**

2. Forward flex
Hold your stomach in and slowly walk your hands down the fronts of your legs to your ankles. Hold for ten seconds, then 'walk' back up to your lap.

3. Foot flex
With your feet flat to the floor, gently roll your soles inwards and outwards. **REPEAT six times.**

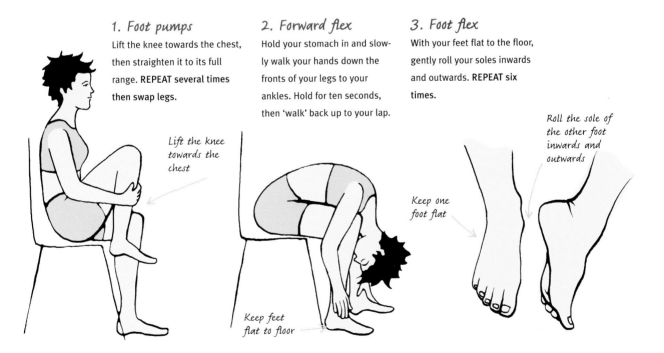

Lift the knee towards the chest

Keep one foot flat

Roll the sole of the other foot inwards and outwards

Keep feet flat to floor

WALK IT OFF

Better legs, better body, better heart: walking is the key
to your exercise regime.

'I walk all the time,' you think. 'I must walk for at least
half an hour each day.' But walking for half an hour a day in
total and walking for half an hour a day in one go are very
different things. To boost fitness levels, you need to be
doing sustained aerobic activity – which means that a
five-minute stroll to the bus stop here and there doesn't
count. It doesn't hurt, but if it's getting fit you want, it
doesn't count either.

WALK TO WORK OUT

If you walk for thirty minutes every other day, you will start
to improve your fitness level in as little as three weeks –
period. However, if it's fat-busting you're after, there are a
few extra tricks you can employ that will really turn your
walk into a proper, fairly strenuous workout. First – and this
one sounds a bit obvious – look straight ahead. Looking
down will slow you down, so keep your neck and shoulders
relaxed, your chin up and your gaze about 4 m (13 feet)
ahead as you walk.

Another fat-burning fact is that the smaller and faster
your steps, the more calories you burn (and also the less
risk of injury you'll face). You can help boost your speed
by remembering to 'lead' with your heels. Correct walking
procedure involves swinging the whole foot forward, land-
ing on your heel, flowing through to the ball of your foot
and then pushing off again with your toes. Finally, to
increase your workout, pump your arms as you go, with
your elbows bent to 90 degrees.

Walking backwards along the street might have one major
drawback – which is that it will win you some strange looks
from passers-by – but it is fabulous for toning the quadriceps and it is also great for improving your balance. You can
rely on your body's own weight to provide the 'resistance'
element in this workout – though don't be tempted to go
down the route of the seriously fitness obsessed and attach
weights to your ankles. This practice can throw out your
normal body alignment. If you do want to add extra resistance while you walk your way to fitness, a weighted
workout vest is the safest option.

'Interval' walking – in other words, speeding up and
slowing down – can also turbo-charge your 'walk-out'.
Over thirty minutes, walk moderately for the first ten, then
step up to a hard walk/easy jog for five, back slightly to a
fast walk for five, back up to an easy jog for five, back down
to a moderate to easy walk for the last five. You can also
intersperse a walk with short bursts of walking on your
heels (great for calves) and toes (for thighs).

For true 'race' walking, you'll need to perfect the 'hip
roll'. As you step your right foot out, push your right hip
forward. Then as the right heel touches the ground, let your
right hip pull your body forward. Finally as your right leg
passes under you, drop your right hip slightly and surge
your left hip forward.

AND STRETCH IT OUT

It's important to stretch out all major muscle groups after
any exercise, even walking – but it's particularly important
to stretch out your legs so as not to risk stiffness and even
swelling in your legs over the next couple of days.

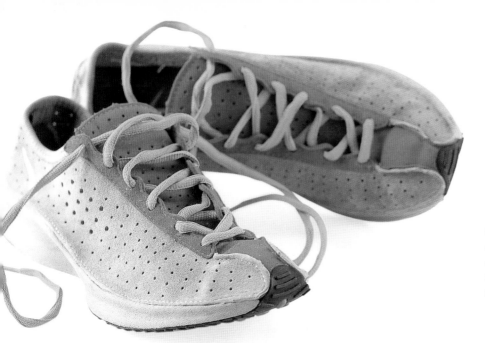

The good news is that stretching out isn't a major time commitment – these three cool-down stretches can be performed in less than a minute. Remember the main pointers: never force a stretch, it should feel good; avoid locking the knees straight; and hold each position for ten to fifteen seconds.

HAMSTRING STRETCH Stand up straight, shoulders down, hips slightly forward. Put one foot up on a chair, platform or anything that will let your leg rest at about 90 degrees to your body. Keep your standing leg soft and gently lean forward from your hips to increase the stretch. Hold and then swap sides.

QUADRICEP STRETCH Stand up straight and have something close by to lean on, like a wall or chair. Bring one foot up to meet your bottom, and clasp it firmly by putting your hand around the 'laces' part of your trainer. Feel the stretch at the front of your thigh. Do the same for the other leg.

CALF STRETCH Using a wall to help, line your feet up against the bottom of the wall and take a step backwards with your left foot. Bend your right knee, using the wall to ensure that the knee doesn't go any further forward than the tip of your right foot. Push the left heel into the floor, and feel the stretch in your left calf. Hold, then swap sides.

After stretching, when you finally hit the shower, pamper your legs a bit: make sure that each of them gets treated to a few minutes under a direct warm spray. This will further relax the muscles and, if you're lucky enough to have a fairly powerful shower, it will even give you a momentary hydrotherapy massage of sorts.

Keep moving about – albeit gently – after your workout and shower to provide further insurance against stiff muscles. However, if at any time you start to feel a bit wobbly or faint, sit down for a few minutes. It could be that the combination of exercise and a warm shower has sent the blood circulation into overdrive, and you will need to give it a few moments to fully settle down.

JUMP TO IT

Now there's no excuse not to work out your legs more often: these exercises are designed to be performed wherever you are.

At home

1. Calf raise and bounce

Stand up straight, holding on to a door handle or chair. Pull yourself up on to your tiptoes then lower yourself all the way down until you're sitting on your heels. Then, when you have reached the ground, bounce on your heels four times. Slowly pull back up to a standing position. Repeat four times. Concentrate on using your legs to do the pushing: don't be tempted to let the door handle take the strain.

2. Single leg raises

Still holding on to the handle, take the leg furthest from the handle and lift it out to the side, pausing in three places on the way up, about 15 cm (6 inches) apart each time, and then again on the way down. As you lift your leg, remember that the third stage is supposed to be the hardest. Swap sides. Repeat each side four times. Keep an eye on your posture throughout: don't lean forward as you lift your leg and put it back down.

Outdoors

3. High skips

This is another good exercise to do when you're out performing your walking exercises. Try skipping for a while instead of walking – it will increase your heart rate and will also give your legs a more strenuous workout. The higher you bring your knees, the more work they will be doing. Even though you will be raising your legs quite high, try to keep the skips fairly close together so that you can fit in the maximum number. If you think 'Scottish Highland dancing', you should get the picture!

4. Bunny hops

You will need about 20–30 m (65–100 feet) of unobstructed grass in order to do this properly. Start on all fours, then jump your feet in so that they're next to your hands, then spring your hands forward another length, bring your feet up to join them and so on. Aim to do around twenty bunny hops. This exercise will also give your arms a bit of a workout, but it shouldn't be attempted if you have weak wrists: if in doubt, jump on the spot or skip instead.

In the gym

5. Leg curl

This exercise works the hamstrings (the muscles situated at the backs of the thighs). Your legs should be fully extended, ankles on top of a cushioned pad and your back at right angles to your legs. Slowly bend your legs so that you're in a normal sitting position, pause, then return your legs to their outstretched staring position. Remember to exhale as you lift the weights and inhale as you lower them. The whole exercise should take around four to six seconds.

6. Leg extension

This works the quadriceps (at the fronts of the thighs). With your ankles secured behind the cushioned pad and toes pointing straight ahead, slowly extend your legs until they are stretching straight out in front of you, hold and then lower them back down. To get maximum benefit, go slowly and exhale as you're lifting your legs up. Do as many reps as you can manage. After two or three sessions, see whether you can slightly increase the 'hold' when your legs are stretched out.

At work — under the desk

7. Leg lifts

Extend one leg so that it is parallel with the other knee. Flex the raised foot, then bounce the raised leg up and down. The smaller the movement, the more effective it will be. Aim for about twenty small bounces, then slowly squeeze the leg back to its original position and swap legs. To target the inner and outer thigh muscles, repeat the exercise but move your leg out to the side and back instead of up and down. For the inner thigh muscles specifically, turn your foot out to the side when you flex it; your ankle should be pointing towards the ceiling.

8. Lower leg stretches

Lift up your leg so that again it stretches straight out in front of you. Imagine you are pulling your foot back in towards your body, so that your heel is the most protruding part and your toes are almost pointing backwards towards your body. This should enable you to feel a strong stretch in your calf; make sure that this is a comfortable stretch for you. Now, keeping that stretch, point your toes forward and count to ten. **REPEAT twice on each leg.**

Stretches — anywhere

9. Yoga downward-facing dog

Position yourself on all fours, your palms flat to the floor, slightly further apart than your shoulders, fingers spread wide. Your feet are on tiptoes. Your spine is arched and your head hangs towards the floor. Feel your spine lengthen and stretch out because of the weight of your head. Now, slowly lower your heels to the floor and feel the stretch all the way down your leg. Taking each foot in turn, lift the heels off the floor and then as it hits the ground again, lift the other foot off simultaneously. Stay like this, or with the heels flat to the floor, for a minute or so, or as long as is comfortable.

10. Yoga dancer's pose

Standing straight, focus on a spot on the wall to help you balance. Lift your right arm, fingers pointing forward, until it is just above shoulder height, and lift your left leg out behind you, as far up as you can, until you can balance easily. It takes practice – focusing on a fixed spot certainly helps.

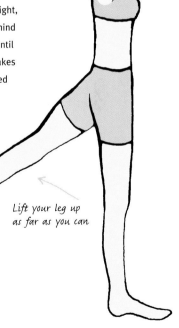

Point your fingers forward

Slowly lower your heels to the floor

Feel the stretch in your legs, back and shoulders

Lift your leg up as far as you can

feather light On days when you want enough energy and vitality to keep you on top

form all day, spare a special thought for your legs. They literally carry you around, so give them an occasional lift

in the form of cooling products, gentle massage or a healthy dose of fake tan.

'LIFT' YOUR LEGS

If there's a start-the-day treatment that's guaranteed to 'lift' your heavy legs, then it's dry body brushing, the microcirculation-boosting routine that's championed by many as the best way to keep the skin smooth. So-called heavy legs are caused in part by sluggish circulation, and the body brushing (or vigorous sweeping of a grainy exfoliating scrub up the legs) will help to eliminate some of the toxins that contribute to this.

Gentle massage will also help. Starting above the knee and working upwards, press, knead and gently pinch your flesh using your thumb and all four fingers. If you're not in a rush, use a massage oil (or plain old olive oil) to help (the oil will take a while to sink in) and put your foot on the edge of a chair or your bed so that you can get to the backs of the thighs.

You can buy special products (usually gels or sprays) to combat heavy legs. They feel heavenly and some are clever-ly formulated to have fast surface evaporation so that they can even be applied through tights. They usually work to stimulate circulation, moisturise and cool legs down. An immediate icy effect might be supplied courtesy of a special synthetic agent that lowers the product's tempera-ture on contact with skin; or it might be through more traditional ingredients such as menthol and eucalyptus.

GOLDEN BRONZE

The glowing, golden colour of a fake tan (also called 'self tan') can do wonders for your legs – and for your self-esteem at the same time. In the same way that we often reach for dark-coloured clothes in order to 'streamline' our figures, a layer of fake tan can make limbs appear more glamorous and svelte.

Booking a one-off salon fake-tanning treatment is not only a great treat, but you can also learn a great deal from your beautician about how best to apply self-tans at home. They'll usually start treatment with a thorough, full-body exfoliation. This will eliminate any dry, scaly patches of skin that the dye will otherwise cling to – leaving you with that unattractive, patchy, 'zebra' look. Unless you have extremely dry skin, it's best then to apply body moisturiser only to particularly rough areas like the knees, ankles and elbows. If you apply body lotion all over, you could create too much 'slip' and make it difficult to rub the fake tan in properly. In salons, it seems that fake tan treatments are becoming ever more high-tech in the quest to banish the appearance of tell-tale streaks. These days you can get your tan airbrushed on, with therapists using airguns that deliver small, super-fine, ultra-natural smatterings of colour that give an even tan, which lasts for three to seven days.

At-home treatments are slightly less space-age, but nevertheless fake tan formulations have come on leaps and bounds since they first came on the scene around a decade ago. However, it's worth noting that whichever type you choose, there are usually trade-offs to be made. For example, as a novice, you will do better to go for a coloured lotion so that you can see where you're going – but these often require a little more waiting time before you can get dressed (usually about fifteen minutes), so most people graduate to colourless lotions when they're a little more experienced. Sprays are the most mess-free option, but coverage is hard to gauge (although some have super-fine spritz nozzles so that the lotion does not have to be rubbed in). While mousses have the advantage of spreading easily, they tend to sink in fast so you might not get the 'slip' you need. For legs, do below the knee first, running the product down the centre of the shin and working out to each side until you meet yourself at the back of the leg. Then do the thigh using the same method. Finally, don't forget to scrub the product from the palms of your hands as soon as you have finished applying it: orange palms are a sure-fire fake-tan giveaway!

Some important fake tan facts to remember: essentially, they are dyes that react with the protein in the skin to form a coloured reaction on the surface. It is possible to build up colour over repeated applications – wait four hours for the 'true' colour to emerge before you re-apply. Contrary to popular belief, the tan provided by a fake tan offers negligible protection against the sun (even a 'real' tan provides only the equivalent of about SPF4). Always wear an SPF15 or higher in the sun, even when you're wearing a fake tan.

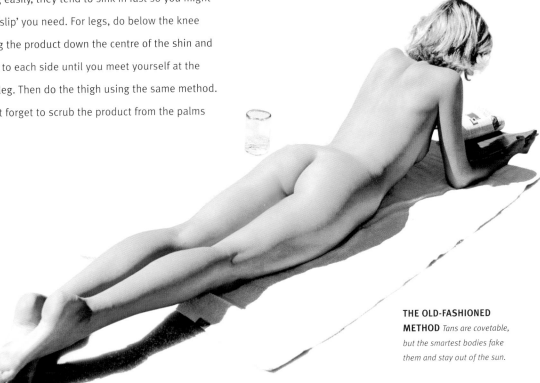

THE OLD-FASHIONED METHOD *Tans are covetable, but the smartest bodies fake them and stay out of the sun.*

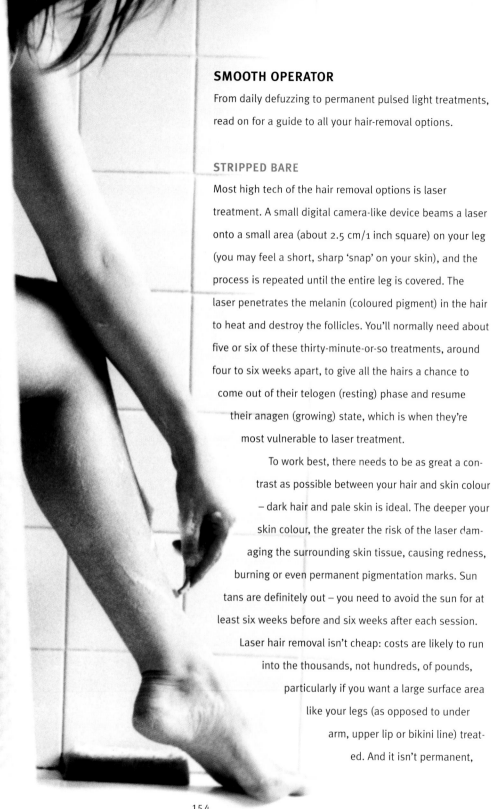

SMOOTH OPERATOR

From daily defuzzing to permanent pulsed light treatments, read on for a guide to all your hair-removal options.

STRIPPED BARE

Most high tech of the hair removal options is laser treatment. A small digital camera-like device beams a laser onto a small area (about 2.5 cm/1 inch square) on your leg (you may feel a short, sharp 'snap' on your skin), and the process is repeated until the entire leg is covered. The laser penetrates the melanin (coloured pigment) in the hair to heat and destroy the follicles. You'll normally need about five or six of these thirty-minute-or-so treatments, around four to six weeks apart, to give all the hairs a chance to come out of their telogen (resting) phase and resume their anagen (growing) state, which is when they're most vulnerable to laser treatment.

To work best, there needs to be as great a contrast as possible between your hair and skin colour – dark hair and pale skin is ideal. The deeper your skin colour, the greater the risk of the laser damaging the surrounding skin tissue, causing redness, burning or even permanent pigmentation marks. Sun tans are definitely out – you need to avoid the sun for at least six weeks before and six weeks after each session. Laser hair removal isn't cheap: costs are likely to run into the thousands, not hundreds, of pounds, particularly if you want a large surface area like your legs (as opposed to under arm, upper lip or bikini line) treated. And it isn't permanent, though it does last longer than other removal methods. Lasers, and their sister treatment, photo-epilation or intense pulsed light, which uses light instead of the laser and has a broader beam to cover a larger area in less time, are approved to offer permanent hair reduction, not removal. With these treatments, there's no guarantee that every last hair will be permanently zapped, and your follicles are also at the mercy of hormonal changes that could restart hair growth later on in life.

Laser hair removal has somewhat outdated electrolysis, which by comparison is painful and slow – each hair has to be treated in turn, whereas lights and lasers can do patches of skin at a time. It's invasive – a needle is stuck into each follicle and an electric current passed through to kill off the hair follicle – and you'll often see redness and irritation immediately afterwards. Permanent hair reduction should, again, be expected only subject to the proviso of other lifestyle factors influencing the results, and though it's probably cheaper than lasers hour for hour, you'll need far more treatments to cover the same area.

DIY OPTIONS

Of the less space-age options, waxing offers slowest regrowth, and unlike shaving, where hairs can grow back stubbly and feel thicker, new hair is actually finer – and after years of waxing, patches of hair can disappear altogether. In salons, a warm wax is applied to the skin so that the hairs are trapped in it. Then strips of fabric are pressed into the wax and ripped off, pulling the hairs out right from the root (hairs need to be at least 3 mm/$\frac{1}{8}$ inch long). At home, you can also get warm waxes, washable strips or ready-prepared disposable cold strips that are less messy but potentially more painful. Any waxing involves some degree of pain. Ways of minimising the discomfort are down to individual trial and error, but it's advisable to steer clear in the week leading up to and during your period, and to make your appointment for the end, rather than the beginning of the day. Finally, if waxing's not for the faint-hearted, it's also not for the weak-skinned. Never wax legs that are sunburned, peeling, chapped or irritated, or have a surfeit of moles, warts or varicose veins.

Good old shaving is the method that most of us revert to for a quick and easy way to remove leg hairs. Its biggest disadvantage is the next-day regrowth and the stubblier hairs (you'll slice off the hair's naturally rounded tip), but the convenience of a quick sweep with the razor followed by instantly silky legs is enough of a draw for most of us. Electric shavers are quick and easy, but they don't often get the same closeness as wet shaving with a disposable razor. These now promise all sorts of technical wizardry, from triple blades to ergonomically designed handles. To avoid irritation, replace them often – at least every three or four outings – and clean thoroughly between uses. To avoid ingrowing hairs (caused when hairs are shaved so short they sit below the skin's surface and grow through skin tissue rather than the hair follicle), always shave hair after soaking in the bath. Shave in the direction of hair growth – just note the way hairs lie when they're flat – and don't reshave areas.

One recent innovation is the growth-inhibiting spritz, which contains vegetal ingredients that slow down the growth of the hair and also make it softer.

vein hopes
Unsightly veins that show through the skin come in all shapes and sizes. You can take measures to avoid broken veins, but these days, there are countless ways in which surgery can help to fade unsightly leg veins away. The question is, do they work – and if so, which one's right for you?

SPIDER VEINS AND VARICOSE VEINS

What makes certain people more susceptible to visible veins (aside from fairer skins) isn't known, but it's thought that pregnancy, heredity and hormonal changes are contributing factors. If you are prone to dilated and swollen veins, don't be surprised to see them cropping up again even after treatments – but hopefully in a much more subdued form. Avoid the problem by losing excess weight and giving up smoking.

Both tiny, red or purple spider veins and larger, blue varicose veins appear when blood vessels dilate so that they sit closer to the skin's surface. The vessels that create spider veins (or telangiectasia) are small capillaries that are tiny to begin with and already lie fairly close to the skin's surface, whereas varicose veins are larger, deeper veins that fill with blood and dilate as a result of faulty valves further inside the body's circulatory system. Unlike spider veins, varicose veins can cause aching – particularly after standing up for prolonged periods – itching and leg swelling.

SURGICAL APPROACHES

Treatments for veins vary, because essentially the same vein could respond differently on different patients. There's normally an element of trial and error involved, and your doctor may feel that one method is better than another in your particular case. This is why, although you can have spider veins treated at beauty salons, it could be best to have them checked over by a doctor first. For example, if varicose veins aren't near enough to the skin's surface, surgical ligation or stripping might be suggested: this involves a general anaesthetic. Incisions will be made to access the vein, which will then be either removed or tied off.

If there is one very long and swollen vein, your doctor might feel that an ambulatory phlebectomy is the best option. Tiny incisions are made all the way along the vein and the surgeon then uses a surgical hook to remove the vein through these little cuts. Although these procedures sound off-putting, it's worth remembering that as surgical procedures go, they are all fairly straightforward.

In most cases, when varicose veins are of average depth and size, sclerotherapy is the first port of call. This is also a common approach to spider veins. It involves injecting the veins with a saline (salt water) substance called sclerosant. This shrinks the veins and then they are reabsorbed into the body and no longer visible from the outside. Usually three to four treatments, involving many injections per session, are needed with a month between each. It's also been shown that wearing compression stockings in between treatments can augment the results

Sclerotherapy

SPIDER veins and varicose veins can be treated with sclerotherapy. Usually three to four treatments are required and a typical treatment lasts from thirty minutes to an hour.

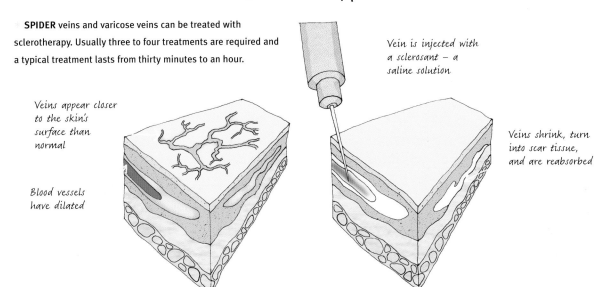

Veins appear closer to the skin's surface than normal

Blood vessels have dilated

Vein is injected with a sclerosant – a saline solution

Veins shrink, turn into scar tissue, and are reabsorbed

by keeping treated veins closed and reducing bruising. Downsides include possible changes in skin pigmentation where the injections were made, and sometimes small blood clots can develop around the injection sites.

TRANSFORMING ENERGY

The main advantage of laser surgery and intense pulsed light therapy is the fact that they can be used deftly to treat more superficial vessels. Lasers and light treatments go under many different brand names, but essentially they all work by beaming an intense wave onto the vein. This is then converted into heat energy, scalding the vein and causing it to wither. In the past there have been problems with pigment in surrounding skin tissue absorbing the waves, resulting in minor burning. This is why fair-skinned women were always

touted as better candidates for laser therapy than those with darker skins. Now, wavelengths and times can be adjusted so that surrounding tissue is not affected, but it is still inadvisable to go for treatments with a sun tan less than six weeks old. You'll normally need between four and eight treatments, each a month apart. Patients describe the laser beam as feeling like an elastic band being snapped against the skin, and the bruising lasts longer than with injections.

A newer-still treatment called Closure is now being championed, too: it's fast, minimally invasive, requires just one treatment and works best on large veins. Tiny incisions are made in the backs of the knees and then a catheter (small tube) is inserted. It bombards the vein wall with radio-frequency energy, which again causes the vein to contract and wither.

LEG SURGERY – THE LONG AND SHORT OF IT

Model-perfect pins that go on forever might be out of the question, but a sexy mini skirt or sporty pair of shorts need not be – find out why.

Many cosmetic procedures are born out of the need to keep up with fashion. And as we all know, models these days are thin, beautiful – and have long, shapely legs. Clothes are increasingly based on the dimensions of these lucky individuals who were born long and lean, while the rest of us have a harder time shopping for jeans and wish enviously for a little of that in-built elegance. Limb-lengthening surgery is not normally performed as a cosmetic procedure in the UK and Europe. It's an extremely lengthy and painful process and is intended only for serious, debilitating skeletal deformities. Nevertheless, when it comes to our legs, other methods of surgery can give nature a little helping hand.

SHAPELY LEGS

One of the most unfair things about legs is that even when the rest of your weight is under control, an otherwise-shapely pair of legs can sometimes be let down by pockets of fat around the knees (particularly the upper tibial area, on the inner side of the leg next to the kneecap), ankles (particularly the lower fibula area, just above the ankle on the outer side of the leg) and calves. Small-volume lipoplasty can work wonders here. The offending fatty deposits can be removed with a syringe or specially shaped cannula through tiny incisions on each side of the Achilles tendon and knee. The smaller the area to be worked on, though, the bigger the room for error – and

the more obvious irregularities can be afterwards. Choose a surgeon who is used to operating on these areas and ask about the techniques that he or she will be using. With the calves, for example, where there is a larger area to work with, lipo-'feathering' is often performed. A little like abdominal etching, it follows the natural contours of the muscles to give a natural appearance, rather than just spot-removing unconnected areas of fat – remember that the legs are a series of intersecting curves. With any lipoplasty of the leg, you must keep your legs elevated for two to three days after surgery, and not shower or bath for a week.

PERFECT CALVES

The calves are another matter. Although it is quite possible to make a difference to your calves through exercise, many people – including body-builders, who often go in for surgery of the calves – find that even their well-toned calves aren't the shape they want. That's where calf implants come in. They're the 'solid silicone' variety as used in the chin, cheeks and buttocks, and are inserted through incisions below the crease behind the knee.

It's a fairly quick procedure – around an hour on each side – and can be carried out under local anaesthetic plus light sedative, as an outpatient. It can be extremely painful for the first week or so afterwards, though, and of course it's difficult to stay off your legs for very long. You need to rest for the first week, and some surgeons recommend that high heels are best worn for a few weeks afterwards in order to take the tension off the calf muscle. In rare cases, the body may reject the implant (as can happen with breast implants) or the implant may weaken the surrounding muscle. Some women find that they get the same 'implant' effect from wearing high heels every day of their lives – although this method is obviously more time-consuming in the long run! Wearing high heels every day can also make a real mess of your feet, crunching your toes and creating corns and calluses.

Our legs are often the site of some of the most obvious genetic similarities within families. If you take after a bulky-legged parent, then there may not be very much that you can do about it. Concentrate on stretching and sculpting exercises, such as Pilates or yoga, in the first instance. Clever dressing can also help. Calf-length skirts that hang midway between the knee and the ankle can help by bisecting bulky calves. Steer clear of shoes and sandals with ankle straps because these can appear to 'cut off' your feet and will disguise the tapering effect at your ankles, which can help to slim down the appearance of your calves.

best foot forward

When we neglect our feet, they let us know it – usually by leaving a bad smell in the air. Here's how changing your diet – and your lifestyle – could help. It's a rare person who can honestly say they've never noticed so much as a slight whiff emanating from the direction of their feet. Whether it's been a hot day, a long day, a hectic day or a scruffy-old-trainers day, the results are often the same: sweaty, smelly feet.

SWEATY FEET

To tackle the sweat issue first, it's worth remembering that you can combat the problem generally, in order to reduce sweating all over the body, or locally by concentrating just on your feet. To combat perspiration as a general problem, there are certain foods you should avoid (no prizes for guessing that garlic, onions and chillis are among them – but see pages 110–11 for a more detailed discussion). If generalised sweating is a problem, visit your doctor. There's a chance it's a symptom of a more serious health problem, such as an overactive thyroid.

When targeting the feet specifically, make time for tea: black tea is good for sweaty feet because it contains tannin, an astringent that will prevent your feet from sweating. Brew five tea bags in a bowl of boiling water and then, when it cools, soak your feet in the bowl for thirty minutes.

AND SO TO SMELL...

Not surprisingly, excessive sweating (hyperhidrosis) and smelly sweat (bromohidrosis) are related to each other. Although the sweat alone doesn't smell, the moisture it provides paves the way for smell-inducing bacteria (most commonly corynebacteria and micrococci) to breed – both on your feet and in your shoes.

In bygone days, shoes were often stuffed with small cotton charcoal-filled bags – the charcoal absorbed oily residue and helped to neutralise smells. These days, odour-absorbing inner soles often still contain charcoal, but their main purpose is to decrease bacteria that are transferred to your feet, not bacteria that are already living in your shoes. By absorbing excess sweat, they'll reduce the moisture problem in your shoes and help that way.

If your shoes are giving off a stench before you even put them on, it could be time they hit the dustbin – or went for a spin in the tumble dryer if they're completely synthetic, like trainers. This won't eradicate the problem indefinitely, but will certainly buy you a bit more odour-free time in which to wear them. The problem with hanging on to smelly shoes is that they will continue to transfer bacteria onto your feet, which in turn could infect your other shoes. Pretty soon all your shoes could be stinking – not a pleasant thought.

Leather shouldn't 'odour up' so easily – it's 'breathable', which means it lets air circulate through it – but even if your shoes are leather, you should wear the same pair only every other day, giving them twenty-four hours to 'dry out' in between.

If you're the kind of person who likes to change into slippers or house shoes when you get home in the evening, think about swapping to a pair of open-toed sandals or flip-flops, which will let more air circulate around your feet. Massaging 'sports' sandals might also be a good idea. Opinion as to whether we should aim to spend a lot of our time barefoot is divided. Some say no, arguing that it is not very hygienic for those who share our living space. Others argue that it is beneficial, and point to the ease with which feet toughen up and become accustomed to even the rockiest terrain. Ultimately, this comes down to your own personal preference. If you like the liberating, 'grounding' feeling of going barefoot, then by all means do it. If you don't, then just be careful not to deny your feet any access to fresh air.

Luckily, nature has a storecupboard full of natural remedies for smelly feet – some more outlandish than others. For example, soaking feet in tomato juice might sound strange but is a good way of neutralising the odour of consistently smelly feet, as is a soak of water, baking soda (a generous sprinkle) and a few teaspoons of cider vinegar. Tea tree oil also crops up in many foot products – it's excellent because it has anti-fungal as well as anti-bacterial properties and has its own enlivening smell, too.

Upping your zinc intake is also a good idea. Increasing your zinc consumption for a few days may help strengthen the skin and make the skin on your feet more resistant to the odour-giving bacteria. Remember to decrease your daily dose in a day or two, though – otherwise your body's absorption of copper could be affected. Also, add anti-fungals to your diet, such as cinnamon, liquorice, coriander, oregano and rosemary.

As a final safety measure, you can also try spraying your feet with some anti-perspirant deodorant before you dress (letting the spray dry first). You don't need a special variety and your underarm product will do just fine. However, inhibiting the effects of bacteria isn't nearly as good as preventing its presence in the first place, so try and eliminate toxins from your diet and see if that works before resorting to anti-perspirant tactics. Again, if all else fails, visit your doctor. He or she can prescribe topical antibiotics, drying solutions and even electric current treatments to discourage perspiration.

flexible friends

Ten thousand steps a day and just twenty-eight little bones to take the strain. It's about time that we paid a little attention to our much-neglected feet. Give your feet a helping hand with the right shoes, moves and exercises.

For most of us, going barefoot equals care-free. It's certainly a good idea to give your feet a chance to breathe every so often, but opinion is divided as to how much time we should spend with nothing on our feet. Some say that wearing breathable slippers or sandals indoors is a good way to avoid cuts and infections, but others hark back to our bare-footed ancestors and point out that feet become hardened when they're constantly exposed, so that you can walk for miles and practically never feel a thing.

SHOPPING FOR SHOES

Whatever – if anything – you wear on your feet indoors, it's not so much of a worry if you wear properly fitting shoes when you're outdoors. Both pregnancy and weight gain can increase foot size, and after the age of around forty the arches in your feet can sometimes begin to fall, causing the foot to flatten and broaden. After this age, try and have your feet measured every year – or whenever you buy a new pair of shoes. Have them measured at the end of the day, when your feet are at their largest, and always standing up.

Remember that the size on the shoe box should be only a starting point. There are no standardised lasts (shoemaker's sizing moulds), so shoe sizes can vary from company to company.

When it comes to buying exercise shoes, the same rules apply. Though trainers are among the best things you can wear on your feet in terms of their 'give' and capacity for shock absorption, it's still unwise to wear them all the time because they are usually manufactured from synthetic materials, and as a result they can often become the breeding ground for some pretty odourous bacteria. You should certainly try not to wear the same pair that you exercise in for your normal activities.

For exercise, don't wear cotton socks – you want fabrics like towelling that draw moisture away from the foot so that you don't slide about, creating blisters, or get athlete's foot infections. But don't let your sports socks be too thin – they can actually let your feet move too much within the shoes and cause blisters. In any case, most modern sports shoes have padding built into the soles.

There are thousands of different types of sports shoes. For top-end athletes, there are important differences, for example, between tennis shoes (superior grip), running shoes (shock-absorbing) and aerobics shoes (lightweight to cushion the ball of the foot), but the rest of us can normally get away with one all-round pair of trainers. Make sure that they have a wide toe box, padded ankle support, laces that extend right up to the bridge of your foot and a cushioned inner sole.

FOOT NOTES

Try the following exercises to increase the strength, flexibility and balance capacity of your hard-working, over-stressed feet.

Flexibility

Ankle circles

Sit on a chair, and extend both your legs out in front of you. Draw circles in the air with your toes. Go both clockwise and anti-clockwise. **REPEAT five times in each direction.**

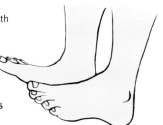

Toe squeezes

Using toe separators (like those for nail polishing) or pen lids between your toes, try and squeeze adjacent toes together, holding for several seconds. **REPEAT five times, mixing up different toes.**

Wobble board

This is a circular piece of wood with a round ball underneath. It's good for flexibility. Make sure you have something close by to hold on to. Roll a 'ball roll' gently forwards and backwards underneath your foot.

Strength

Toe grabs

Sit on a chair with a towel or thick cloth on the floor. Scrunch your toes up in order to pick up the cloth and lift it off the floor. Repeat five times. Also try picking up marbles and dropping them into a bowl.

Toe raises

Have your heels in the air and the balls of your feet and toes resting on a thick book. Slowly lower your heels to the floor and then raise yourself again, and hold for ten seconds. **REPEAT fifteen times.**

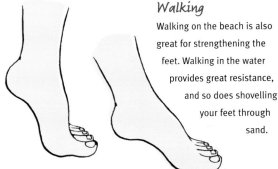

Walking

Walking on the beach is also great for strengthening the feet. Walking in the water provides great resistance, and so does shovelling your feet through sand.

Balance

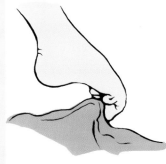

Heel walks

Just as the name suggests, lift your toes off the floor and walk along, just on your heels. Get as high up on your heels as you possibly can, keeping your legs straight. Try and take ten steps with each foot clockwise.

Line walks

Find a completely straight line – for example, the line where two paving stones meet – and then walk along it sideways, crossing one foot over the other. Do two 'crossovers' one way, then back again.

Tai chi

As well as being great for relaxing and improving concentration, this is an excellent form of exercise for those wishing to improve foot balance because it works on grounding the body, improving posture and learning how to sway.

sole survivor

When we talk about neglected feet, we're usually talking about dry, scaly and generally tired-looking (and -feeling!) feet. The fact is that looking after the skin on your feet isn't the same as looking after the skin on your body – although most of us presume it is. For a start, feet need extra attention when it comes to keeping them clean and dry.

A GUIDE TO COMMON FOOT PROBLEMS

Athlete's foot is a fungus and, like most fungal infections, thrives in warm, damp conditions. It's also notoriously difficult to get rid of. When you've had a bath or shower, take a clean, designated 'foot towel' and dry thoroughly in between every toe. Only when your feet are totally dry – at least ten minutes later – should you treat with an anti-fungal cream or powder.

The skin on your soles is also thicker than the skin on your body, and heels in particular become parched and can appear rough and dry. Taking baths, not showers, helps soften hard skin, and so long as the skin's not broken, a vigorous rub with a pumice or foot file while skin is still soft will work wonders. If your heels have become so dry that you've got cracked skin, heal the cracks with an antiseptic and use an unscented moisturiser twice daily.

If you've got particularly sweaty feet, it's important not to overmoisturise. In fact, keeping feet baby soft can actually cause problems if you don't wear properly fitting shoes: if they're too big, the foot can slide about, and if they're too small, they can be easily pinched together. Both of these scenarios can lead to calluses. They're layers of skin that build up so as to protect the foot from further damage – but the fact that we're constantly putting pressure right on top of them means that the older layers often aren't shed regularly enough, so the skin becomes tough and could eventually turn into a corn.

Corns are calluses that develop on the tops of the toes. When your shoes press on them it can be very painful. Corns are more common as we age because the foot's layer of fat diminishes, and while calluses and smaller corns can usually be removed by daily filing with a foot file, larger ones often need the help of a chiropodist. You can buy special pads that stick over the corn to cushion it. Some are medicated to gradually soften the hard, leathery skin.

Another, more serious consequence of toe-cramping shoes is a bunion. This deformity that develops at the base of the big toe can cause a great deal of pain, interfere with walking properly and distort the entire foot in a way that is decidedly unattractive. It gets progressively worse over time, so if the side of your foot near your big toe is only slightly red and only slightly swollen, it's not too late to change your taste in shoes. Discard any that prevent your toes from lying flat and pointing forward, and even spreading a bit when you walk. If you let a bunion worsen, you are increasing the risk of developing osteoarthritis in the toe joint later in life, and probably heading towards bunion surgery. This procedure involves cutting through the skin to the bone, cutting back the bony overgrowth and realigning the toes. It is done under general anaesthesia, may involve a hospital stay and will be followed by a recovery of up to six weeks, during which time you must wear an ungainly surgical sandal. Most often, each foot is done separately so you can at least hobble about while you're recovering. That's a lot of pain and trouble for the sake of a sexy pair of shoes!

CHECK YOUR REFLEXES

Massaging your feet can have untold benefits for the rest of the body. Reflexology is a form of natural therapy that involves massaging the feet principally but sometimes the hands as well. The premise of reflexology is that the whole body can be divided into ten zones, each zone having a corresponding 'reflex' area on the foot. Massaging the different areas of the feet and unblocking trapped energy flows can have positive effects on the rest of the body, too.

Reflexology is one of the most popular of all the natural healing therapies. Many who go for treatments have no specific complaints but relish the feeling of energy that this natural treatment gives them. Advocates say that by isolating areas of malfunctioning energy flow in certain parts of the body, reflexology can help draw attention to potential areas of trouble and encourage prevention of more serious conditions.

It's fair to say that most devotees of reflexology already have ailments that they wish to work on. Reflexology's aim is to help the body to heal itself, and the conditions that it claims to be particularly beneficial for include arthritis, back pain, digestive complaints, insomnia, migraines, sinus problems and stress. One of the best things about reflexology is that you can practise certain of the elements yourself. For migraines, for example, gently squeezing the tops of your big toes can help, and for shoulder tension, massaging the bean-shaped patch of flesh on the edge of the feet, below the big toe, can bring relief.

Reflexology points

Top of head/brain   Pituitary   Sinuses

Side of head/brain   Neck   Ears

Eyes   Thyroid

Eustachian tube   Heart

Shoulder   Solar plexus   Stomach

Pancreas

Lung   Stomach   Spleen

Diaphragm   Pancreas   Waist

Liver   Kidney

Gall bladder   Bladder   Small intestine

Ascending colon   Rectum

Ileo-caecal valve   Sciatic nerve

REFLEXOLOGY involves the application of pressure to various reflex areas (mainly on the soles of the feet) to promote energy flow and treat health problems.

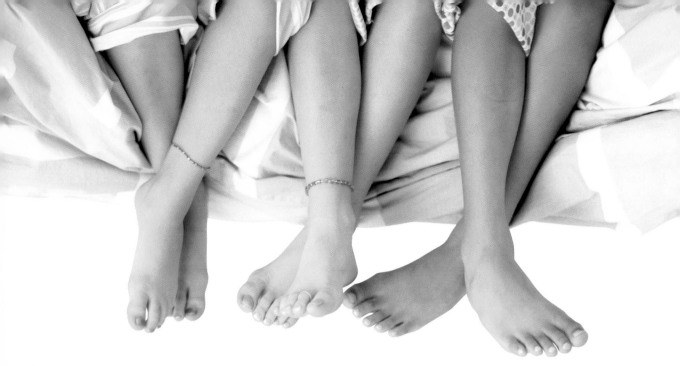

PERFECT THIRTY-MINUTE PEDICURE

If you don't have time to go to the salon, don't despair. You can have your feet primed, polished and ready to party in the time it takes to watch your favourite soap.

SCRUB, SALT AND SOAK: TEN MINUTES

First, lay out a towel for your feet and sit a large bowl of warm water by it. Remove any old nail polish. Take a teaspoon's worth of exfoliator for each foot and rub it in. Remember that the thing about scrubs is to sweep them along, not work them into the surface of the skin. Cover both the underside and tops of feet.

Next, add a softening ingredient to the water. You can buy special 'foot soaks', but you can also make your own very easily with ordinary storecupboard ingredients such as powdered milk, almond oil or even plain old table salt.

A few drops of relaxing essential oil wouldn't go amiss either – just choose your favourite. Immerse your feet and loosen the exfoliating grains with your fingers. Soak for around five minutes, then pat feet dry with a fluffy towel, making sure you remove any remaining scrub and drying well between the toes.

RUB, REVIVE AND REPAIR: TEN MINUTES

Once your feet are dry, take a foot file or pumice stone and give feet a good rub in all the dry spots such as heels, balls of the feet and outsides of the soles. Now apply a super-rich moisture cream to those same areas, really rubbing it in until a thick (i.e., visible) layer of cream has disappeared.

Now for the nice and relaxing bit: the foot massage. Sit with one foot brought up to the middle, and apply a few drops of massage oil. Taking your foot in both hands, use your thumbs to massage the soles of your feet, paying particular attention to your instep. Massage each toe in turn by rubbing it between your fingers and then gently pulling on it before releasing. If you like, continue massaging right up your calves.

While your feet are nice and soft, it's time to tidy up your cuticles. If you're confident, you can buy special AHA creams that help dissolve cuticles. If not, add a drop of oil to each cuticle and gently push each one back with the edge of a rounded cuticle tool. While you're doing this, check the underside of your toenails and with a tissue remove any excess oil or lotion that's settled down there.

SHAPE, SHINE AND SHIMMER: TEN MINUTES

To cut your toenails, take a pair of nail clippers and cut straight across the tops of your nails. This part is simply about getting the right length – most people tend to go for a shortish length with a small white edge, but if you're a sporadic pedicurist, it might be better to go short and give your nails room to grow.

Next, take a nail file and round off the edges. Straight-edged toenails can result in ingrowing toenails that may become infected and painful, whereas rounded edges cannot penetrate the skin so easily. As with fingernails, file in one direction only and wipe flakes from each toenail after filing or they will get trapped under the polish.

Professional pedicurists often buff nails before polishing. This adds a shine to natural nails and also creates a smooth, clean surface that nail polish can glide easily along. Invest in a nail file that has a 'buffing' surface on one of its flat sides. Next, apply a transparent base coat – it's

particularly important if you're going for a dark nail colour that could stain your nails. Leave it to dry for around a minute before applying your colour.

Shake your nail polish bottle well and rub it between both your hands to warm it slightly and get rid of any gloopiness. Wipe off excess polish from the front and back of the brush and then rest the brush in the middle of the nail, about 2 mm/$\frac{1}{14}$ inch above the cuticle – as you press the brush down, it will naturally cover this extra bit. Now fill in the polish at either side of the middle 'stripe', using it as a guide.

Apply two coats of your chosen colour, then finish off with another coat of transparent polish. 'Top coats' and 'base coats' are pretty much interchangeable; base coats tend to be thicker, whereas top coats will dry faster. Don't worry about using the same product before and after nail colour.

Pedicure checklist

✳ **FOR** salon-style foot pampering at home, here's all the kit you need for a perfect pedicure.

Scrub, salt and soak NEED towel, bowl of warm water, nail varnish remover and cotton wool, exfoliating scrub, foot soak

Rub, revive and repair NEED foot file, moisture cream, massage oil, cuticle remover, cuticle oil, rounded cuticle tool, tissues

Shape, shine and shimmer NEED nail clippers, nail file, base coat, nail polish, top coat

feet first

Are you sandal-shy? Do you love your stilettos but hate your feet? If you are unhappy with the actual shape of your toes, then no amount of pedicures, no matter how pampering, is going to help. If you're prepared to go the long haul in pursuit of glamorous feet, surgery could make a difference.

DIVIDED OPINIONS

The issue of foot surgery causes serious divisions between many medical experts. Most podiatrists (foot doctors) say that feet are very complicated and intricate (with over 24 different bones), and are far too important in our daily lives to take the risk of operating for purely aesthetic reasons. Some cosmetic surgeons take a different view, arguing that being unhappy with your feet is no different from being unhappy with your nose, for example – particularly for women who want to be able to wear fabulous sandals – and that cosmetic surgery is permissible for this reason.

COMMON PROCEDURES

One of the most common cosmetic procedures performed on the feet is to shorten the second toe when it is longer than the big toe. The fact is that this can be seen as both a medical and a cosmetic treatment – depending on your motivation. Some people simply don't like the look of it and can also find it difficult to get shoes to fit. But for some people, the longer toe takes the brunt of their weight when they walk, causing it to bend or buckle at the joint and forming hard skin or calluses at the tip.

A small incision is made at the top or side of the toe, and a tiny piece of bone is clipped away so that it corresponds to one or more of the other toes. Bandages will be worn for a week afterwards and walking will feel strange at first, but it normally takes only a few weeks to get used to the new arrangement. It's better to wear flat shoes at first.

Podiatrists also complain that the high-heeled shoes so beloved by many women make their feet worse, making surgery necessary. So-called hammer toes, where the tip of the toe points downward rather than lying flat, fall into this category – although in fairness to stiletto wearers, most 'hammer toes' are due to congenital defects or injuries, not unkind footwear. Surgery is the last resort. You'll probably be advised to try padding and shoe inserts, and anti-inflammatory medication (including cortisone shots) to relieve the pain. Of course, none of that will make your toe look normal, so if it's a better-looking foot you're after, surgery may be able to get it to straighten out and lie down. The skin and blood supply in the toes can be stretched by no more than 6 mm ($\frac{1}{4}$ inch), so toe-lengthening procedures wouldn't work for seriously short or crooked toes. As with bunion surgery, the recovery time can be lengthy.

An incision is made at the tip of the toe and a tiny silicone implant inserted. It can take some getting used to, and bandages will have to be worn for around ten days, making walking difficult. The other major drawback could be that the implants can often look quite obvious owing to the fact that the toes don't have large quantities of fat to disguise them. On the other hand, even a small 'ripple' where the implant lies may be preferable to crooked toes – and will probably stand out less.

HIGH HEELS

It's clear that as far as some women are concerned, high heels will never go out of fashion. But no-one ever said they were comfortable. That's why the latest – and one of the most extreme – procedures in the foot surgery arena involves putting synthetic implants into the ball of the foot, raising it up slightly and providing a 'cushion' for the foot so as to give the foot better 'balance' and protection when wearing high-heeled shoes.

This procedure is still in the early stages of development, and there are obvious concerns about implants leaking and moving in an area in which they are going to be subject to so much wear and tear. However, the level of interest being displayed in the procedure is testament both to our apparently unceasing love of high heels, and also to our receptivity to surgical solutions for common aesthetic problems.

BONES OF CONTENTION
Some experts think that the feet should not be operated on without good reason.

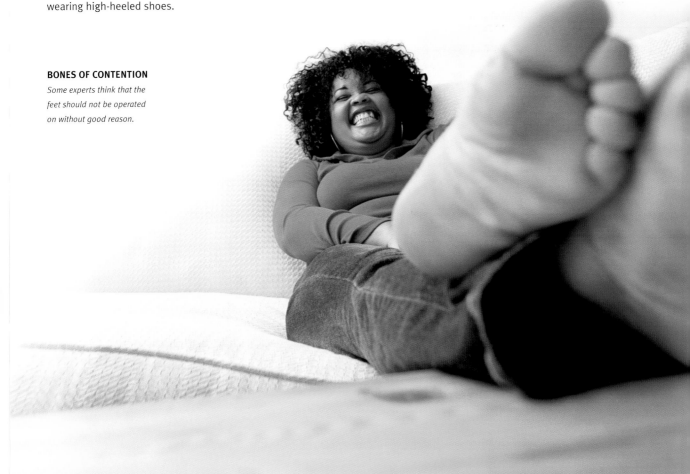

what is my motivation? Most diet and fitness plans take a nosedive in less than a week. Make yours stick by finding out the motivating tricks that will really work for you. The good news is that the best ways don't involve life-changing routines: just small, easy alterations. You won't just be able to fit these into your day: you'll actually want to.

REASONS FOR RELUCTANCE

To find your motivation, first identify your usual excuse. For some people, time is a pressure and moreover, they simply don't enjoy exercise. The last thing they want to do is use up precious free time doing boring old sport. If this is you, make your reluctance your motivation and find ways to slip some fitness benefits into your normal activities.

One good trick is for a week, do anything and everything that involves movement – walk up the stairs instead of using the lift, walk rather than drive to the supermarket, park away from the supermarket doors. Don't measure how far you've walked, or calculate how much time you've spent doing it, just carry on making all those minute changes to your day. Soon they will start to become habitual.

Habit is good for anyone who finds it hard to stick to a fitness routine because – and here's the clever bit – it won't feel like you're making any special effort. Walking up the stairs, choosing the furthest parking space, will just be the things you do normally. Once you've increased your general fitness levels like this, you'll actually feel like walking small distances rather than driving in the future, anyway.

So what if you're the sort of person who has good intentions, but bottles them when you get halfway to the gym/to the front of the sandwich queue? Chances are you're the all-or-nothing type and think half an hour in the gym is little more than a drop in your fitness ocean. Try massaging your ego with the 'visualisation' technique.

On the way to the gym, visualise how fantastic you'll feel when you've finished your workout: not just physically, but how pleased you'll be that you managed to make time for a workout. You can also imagine how frustrated you'll be with yourself if you don't go... But don't dwell on the negatives for too long – just long enough to get you through the door and onto the treadmill! Visualise yourself with the fab new pair of shoes you've promised yourself when you reach your first target, and visualise yourself at that friend's wedding in a few months when you'll have lost inches all over.

Finally, if you're basically happy with your shape, your health should be your motivation. Half an hour's aerobic exercise on most days of the week is proven to reduce your odds of heart disease, osteoporosis and a variety of other life-threatening conditions. Plus it's not just you who will feel the difference – think of all the other people who will benefit from you being happy and energetic – kids, parents, partner, friends, colleagues.

Your golden rule is to plan ahead. Make a commitment to take a yoga class next Wednesday, and arrange to see a friend there: two fail-safe reasons to ensure you turn up.

WHAT DO I DESERVE?

Rewards are good. Rewards are helpful. In fact, not to put too fine a point on it, rewards are entirely necessary. What they shouldn't be is off-putting. It's no good losing 10 lbs (4.5 kilos) and then rewarding yourself with a big cream cake that you immediately feel guilty about. Rewarding yourself with a calorie-laden treat is tantamount to saying, 'This is to remind me of what I'm missing.' You should concentrate on those things that you are gaining – a healthier lifestyle and more confidence. So why not just have the cream cake anyway, guilt-free, and then move on? No diet is about denying yourself all the time.

Your new way of living shouldn't be a strict regime that you're forcing yourself to live by until you've reached your desired goal. It should be an attitude, a new approach. As you begin your new approach to your body, your rewards should be things that have a direct bearing on whatever you've achieved. If you're on a weight-loss programme, try on some outfits that are normally a bit tight, and see how much better they fit.

If you're stepping up your fitness routine, treat yourself to a new workout top – there's no better way to get you into the gym. A new CD to exercise to? Get your skin as ship-shape as your body with a couple of hours of 'home spa', complete with candles, bubble bath and glossy magazines.

And what about sharing your achievements with someone else? You might prefer to keep your goals to yourself – and that's absolutely fine – but there's certainly no harm in mentioning that you've started walking thirty minutes a day and are feeling much fitter as a result. Basking in someone else's admiration can work wonders for your motivation – and your self-esteem.

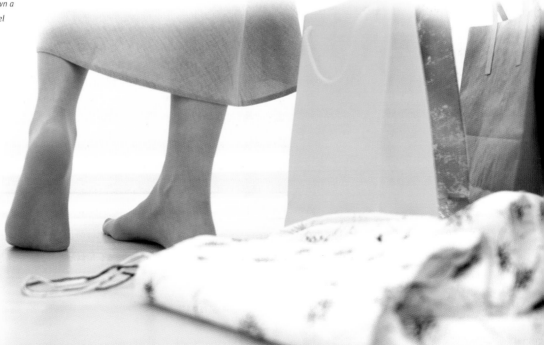

RETAIL THERAPY *There's nothing like dropping down a dress size to make you feel like hitting the shops.*

stir it up
You're over the first flush of enthusiasm, and you've hit a motivational dry patch. Spice up your workout programme with a bit of variation. It may not seem like it at first, but there are hundreds of fitness-related activities that you could be doing, and who knows? You might actually end up enjoying some of them!

CHOP AND CHANGE

It's good to make a habit of exercise, but it's bad to get into exercise habits. This may sound contradictory, but what it means it this. While it's true that you need to set regular time aside for exercise, when you're actually working out, it's important to mix up what you do. If you're looking for all-round body improvement, then sticking to the same machines in the gym, running the same two-mile course or swimming the same thirty laps simply won't cut it.

MIXING IT...

This simple principle is known in the fitness world as 'cross training' – it basically means mixing up your exercise routine so that you're not constantly exercising the same old muscle groups (as you would if you were using only an exercise bike, or jogging every day). It also distributes the impact that you load on to certain parts of the body (for example, on your ankles when jogging or your arms when using free weights), thus reducing your risk of muscle overload and injury.

Unless you're competing for a certain event or are determined to build up one set of muscles particularly, cross training is possibly the best form of exercise to go in for. Another of its advantages is that it often lets you keep training even if you've got an injury, because you can simply concentrate on other parts of the body. Also, it's a well-known fact that for most people, routine equals chore. If you always go swimming on Wednesdays, don't – go jogging instead. The new surroundings and new set of challenges will give you a different perspective on your fitness levels (maybe you'll be able to jog further than last time you tried), plus when you hit the pool again, you won't feel so beholden to it, meaning your boredom/frustration levels will diminish.

Remember that your whole routine is all about choice. If you don't feel like leaving the house today, stick on an exercise video and away you go. Including an exercise video in your fitness routine every once in a while can be fantastic for relieving boredom – it's only when you start seeing the same one day after day that you feel like throwing it out of the window. See the chart opposite for some exercise ideas.

CALL IN THE EXPERTS

But what if you've been exercising for what seems like ages and not seeing any results, or what if your original achievements have now 'plateaued' and you don't know how to jump to the next level? A personal trainer could be

Cross-training chart

✱ **VARYING** your workouts means there's less chance of getting bored and giving up. Use this chart as a basis for your own programme.

Monday	Tuesday	Wednesday	Thursday	Friday	Saturday	Sunday
brisk walking 30 mins	weight training (upper body) 30 mins	swimming 30 mins	brisk walking, cycling 30 mins	weight training (lower body) 30 mins	jogging/brisk walking 30 mins	yoga/stretching 30 mins
	stretching 5 mins	yoga 30 mins	stretching 10 mins			

just what you need. They're not a new breed, but their surge in numbers has meant that it's now possible for everyone to have access to one. Some gyms employ 'in-house' trainers, who can be consulted as part of your membership, but most trainers have a fairly steep hourly rate.

One of the most helpful things about seeing a personal trainer is that it ties you down to a time and place. And you can go through the motions without having to worry about whether or not you're doing the right thing – your trainer will take care of all that. But unless you're the sort of person who won't get motivated without someone standing over them, see a trainer as you'd see your dentist – for regular check-ups or if you feel something's wrong.

The biggest hurdle is finding a trainer who you like and trust. They should come if possible by referral – through a friend or your gym, for example, or even from an organisation like the National Register of Personal Fitness Trainers (*see* Contacts). Even when you're only talking basic fitness, a skilled trainer should be trained in

anatomy, physiology, injury prevention and first aid. As you work out a fitness programme together, expect your trainer to explain to you why you're doing each exercise and what benefits it has. If he or she doesn't do this, just ask.

Seeing a personal trainer can be daunting. Even if we trust our trainers, many of us still end up embarrassed about our weight/fitness/aptitude. Don't be. You wouldn't expect your dentist to laugh at you if you needed a tooth out, or your mechanic to laugh when your car broke down. Good personal trainers just want to help increase your fitness and boost your confidence – and remember, they've almost always seen a lot worse than you.

Another spin on the personal trainer approach is to organise personal training sessions with a group of friends. This is particularly enjoyable for people who enjoy race-type activities or who are just competitive by nature. Many people find that comparing their fitness levels with a companion forces them to increase their concentration levels and provides extra motivation.

get well, stay happy

Mood-enhancing treatments are the latest way to relax your body and uplift your mind. From the obvious (like taking a bath) to the outrageous (such as laughter therapy), there are dozens of ways to reduce your tension levels, lift your mood and even express yourself. All you have to do is find the one that suits you best, then relax and enjoy.

WATER THERAPY

Ever emerged from a warm bath feeling as if the day's stresses have just floated away? Hydrotherapy (water treatment) and hydrothermal therapy (water plus temperature treatment) have been around since Roman times, but are now re-emerging as safe, effective ways to treat the symptoms of diseases and also calm and relax the mind. They're particularly useful in the treatment of joint pain, arthritis, lower back pain and insomnia.

The theory is that by applying different water pressures and temperatures to the nerve endings, impulses are carried deeper into the body, where they can stimulate the immune system, invigorate the circulation and digestive systems, decrease pain sensitivity and diminish stress hormone production.

Treatments can take the form of baths, showers, wraps and rubs. Warm water soothes, while cold invigorates. To stimulate circulation, you might be given a shower that alternates warm with cold water – especially good for arthritis of the hands and feet.

Most day spas offer hydrotherapy treatments, but you can also self-treat at home. For a treatment to relieve back pain, try a 'back douche': with your shower spray on its lowest setting (so that the water runs onto your skin without splashing back), let warm water rain directly on your back for several minutes. Then stroke off excess water, dress and do some gentle exercise.

LAUGH IT OFF

Another form of mood-lifting therapy is laughter therapy. It's described as 'meditation without the concentration' because its advocates say it provokes an absence of conscious thought similar to meditation. Its main advantage, unsurprisingly, is its capacity for stress relief, but the knock-on benefits are thought to be great. It's reputed to help high blood pressure and heart disease sufferers particularly, but it can also assist people with breathing complaints stemming from bronchitis and asthma: laughter improves lung capacity and oxygen levels in the blood.

For a serious bout of laughter, laughter clubs are now springing up regularly, and the infectious nature of getting the giggles can mean that it's much easier to laugh in a crowd than on your own. Having said that, try settling down in front of a video of your favourite comedian (but keep the laughs coming fast and furious – it's thought that fifteen minutes' sustained laughter a day is the optimum for health and wellbeing benefits).

MOOD BOOSTERS

Light therapy is now becoming an important way for the millions who suffer from seasonal affective disorder (or SAD – depression and reduced vitality due to lack of exposure to daylight) to make it through the long winter months. It's four times more prevalent in women than men, and doesn't just affect moods: it can also increase your appetite, up your sleep requirement so that you're more lethargic and affect your propensity for movement and exercise, so that weight may increase and fitness levels drop.

Research suggests that the brighter the light, the better we feel – although the reasons for this aren't yet properly understood by scientists. Artificial lights normally give us a lux count of between 250 and 1,000, whereas sunlight can exceed 20,000. This explains why most light therapy takes the form of special full-spectrum 'light boxes' that can mimic sunlight at home or in your office: ordinary artificial lights simply aren't strong enough. Doctors can prescribe a course of treatment for you – most range from either a short burst of intense light (for example, thirty minutes at 10,000 lux) to up to two hours at a lower intensity (around 2,500 lux). Patients usually say that they notice a difference within a week of commencing treatment. It's also important to get outside as often as possible – at lunchtimes, for example – and make sure you look up and around as you walk.

One of the easiest mood-boosting therapies to practise at home is nutritional therapy. Start with a good multivitamin, then make sure you eat foods that help your hormones and nervous system. Without adequate levels of Omega-3 fatty acids in the nervous system, for example, you're more vulnerable to depression, so eat more oily fish. Also, avoid anything sugary that gives you a 'quick lift', then brings you back down when the effects wear off – steady blood sugar levels are the key to 'happy' food. Caffeine is also guilty of this kind of mood dipping – try drinking mood-relaxing St John's Wort tea instead. Other good herbal remedies include lavender, lemon balm, linden blossom, ginseng and rosemary.

Finally, step up your supplies of foods that contain the amino acid tryptophan – it's involved in producing the mood-enhancing neurochemical serotonin. It's found in lean poultry, bananas, almonds, cottage cheese and dairy products. These foods may not have you leaping up and down with joy, but by lifting your serotonin levels slightly you increase your chances of achieving an even emotional keel – and this is surely the ultimate aim for all of us.

UPLIFTING *As you get your body into shape, remember to consider your emotions and state of mind.*

now you try

One of the first steps towards building yourself a better body involves feeling better about yourself – and that can come only from within. Use this ten-point plan to think, feel and act more confident so that you're ready to take charge of your life – today.

1. Positive thinking

We are constantly engaged in a dialogue with our own thoughts. If you're feeling bad about yourself, what you're actually doing is feeling bad about what your thoughts are telling you. So don't hate them – change them. Tell yourself positive things instead. If you can keep it up for twenty-four hours, you'll be well on the way.

2. The 'equal time' rule

If you're finding positive thoughts hard to come by, try the 'equal time' rule. For every minute you spend dwelling on something about your body that you don't like, spend equal time considering something about yourself that you are pleased with. My thighs wobble – but my feet are cute. I'm a bit overweight – but my new haircut takes years off me.

3. Keep it real

When you're frustrated at something you've done, especially if it's something like letting your diet lapse or gym programme slide, remember that you're human, not perfect and that doing well isn't about never putting a foot wrong. Celebrities with model-perfect figures don't live in the real world. They have beauticians, personal trainers and chefs to keep them in line. Never feel guilty for being who you are – just start each day afresh.

4. Taking charge

Confidence is about knowing who you are and accepting the good and the bad. This means taking responsibility for your actions. A good way of deciding what to do is to ask yourself: 'What's my motivation here?' When you know what's driving you to do something, you can make decisions that are based on achieving that goal.

5. Beauty boosters

As well as getting confidence from accomplishing your goals, you will thrive on affirmation from others. Quick-fix beauty solutions can give you an extra boost (*see pages 183–84*). When you're going out, spend time getting ready so that you look and feel your best. If you've skipped anything, your anxieties will jump on it.

6. Use your imagination

Just because you're not feeling confident doesn't mean other people can tell. But if you're worried that you don't have any confidence and your anxieties will show through – fake it. Imagine you're playing a part – a fantastic party hostess, a self-assured interview candidate, whatever. It might even help to think of a fantastic real-life role model or character in a movie. What words would you use to sum them up? Now become those characteristics yourself.

7. Confidence, not arrogance

Don't worry that people will mistake confidence for arrogance. Arrogance is a belief that you know more than other people – confidence is when you know yourself. Being truly confident means letting everyone have their say – something you'll never find arrogant people doing.

8. Challenge yourself

We become nervous when we feel like a 'spare part'. If you feel like this at a party or function, try to give yourself a task to achieve. It might be finding out whether you like the people you're with; fact finding or gaining business contacts; learning to improve a certain skill; or meeting as many new people as you can. We thrive on challenges, and even if it's just a silly test, it will help you forget your nerves.

9. Boost your mood

Have an arsenal of quick fixes that will instantly boost your mood – favourite songs, a particular friend or relative you can call, photos of holidays and so on. If you're feeling low, call on one of these: you can 'train' yourself to feel good when you want.

10. Knowledge is power

If you are unhappy with your body shape, learn about how to make changes. There's nothing like knowledge to boost your confidence. Arm yourself with facts about food and exercise.

BOOST YOURSELF *There are lots of easy ways to improve your confidence levels and generally feel better about yourself.*

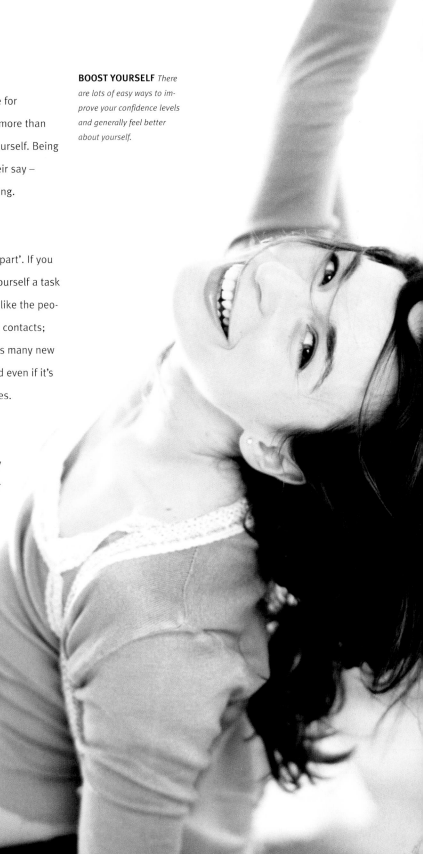

spring clean your body

So now you've begun to clear out those self-confidence cobwebs – make sure your body's in great shape, too. The best way to start is by giving your body a good old spring clean – detoxing isn't easy, but the results are well worth the effort.

HEALTH CRAZE

'Detoxing' is one of the biggest crazes in the health and beauty industry at the moment, and it encompasses everything from trendy juice diets to 'detoxifying' massage oils and bubble baths. As with any such bandwagon, the core principle is to be applauded – but there's a lot of hype to cut through in order to get down to the simple facts.

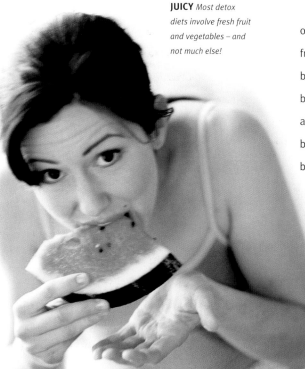

JUICY *Most detox diets involve fresh fruit and vegetables – and not much else!*

TOXIC OVERLOAD

The word 'detoxification' literally means 'eliminating toxins (poisons)'. In the high-tech world we live in, we're surrounded by chemicals that bombard our skin, hair and respiratory and digestive systems – in fact, every single part of our bodies. From pollution to pesticides, prescription drugs to plastic containers, we've never had so much direct contact with chemicals as we do now.

Of course, our bodies weren't designed to process any of these artificial substances and, as a result, we can suffer from toxic overload, resulting in a build-up of toxins in our bodies. The most common signs of a chemically overloaded body include grey skin, dull hair and sluggish energy levels, although other conditions such as stress, asthma, irritable bowel syndrome and allergies can all be brought on by toxin build-up. Some doctors even blame years of toxin build-up for the onset of some degenerative diseases in later life. They believe that embarking on regular detox programmes can boost your immune system and help fight infection as it arises.

In theory, what detoxification does is clear out as many of the built-up toxins as possible. There are a variety of ways in which it can be done, although most detox programmes centre on stripping the diet back to the very basics for anywhere between two days and a month. There are many differing opinions about how long a detox programme needs to be in order to have a worthwhile effect, but it's generally agreed that ten-day programmes can make significant improvements without seriously affecting your lifestyle. It's also debatable how often you should detox – although if you could plan to do it once or twice a year, your body would certainly reap the benefits

THE DETOX DIET

Most detox programmes suggest beginning with a twenty-four-hour fast. This means nothing passes your lips except water (bottled or filtered, not from the tap), so you need to pick a day when you can relax at home – but banish food from temptation's way before you begin! It's helpful to bear this in mind the day before – not by overcompensating and stocking up on calorie-laden goodies, but by cutting out stimulants such as coffee and tea and avoiding carbohydrate-heavy meals.

The next day, you begin the detox diet proper. Your raw ingredients will mostly be....raw. Fresh fruit – particularly apples, grapes, pineapple and watermelon, plus fresh raw vegetables (although not potatoes). Mineral water should still be your main drink – take it with a slice of lemon for flavour – and instead of drinking coffee or black tea, try herbal teas known for their detoxifying properties, such as elderflower and dandelion.

This will be your list of 'allowed' foods for the next week. Don't expect to feel fabulous straightaway – you'll probably feel exhausted, hungry and even tearful until around day four. Then things will start to get easier –

particularly as you'll probably be spurred on by a brighter complexion, shinier eyes and of course a looser waistband! (Detox-diet weight loss isn't permanent, though – most of what is lost is water.) On days nine and ten, start introducing other 'clean' foods into your meals, such as fish, brown rice, olive oil and soya milk.

In order to spur you on even further, supplement your nutritional detox with some beauty treatments, too. While your liver is doing most of the work within your body, the skin is the route out of the body for many of the toxins, so it's important to keep your cell renewal process up to scratch. Daily dry body brushing is a fabulous way to do this – it will rid the skin of those dead cells that are clinging to the surface.

If that sounds a bit energetic, go for the 'reward' option and treat yourself to a massage – or at the very least, a massage oil that you can use on yourself. Best for detox will be those with essential oils of grapefruit, orange, ginger, lemon and bergamot – add a few drops to your bath, too, to really kick-start your circulation. Leave yourself time for the oils to really sink in, too – after all your hard detoxing work, you deserve the treat.

For an internal approach, try a colonic treatment. The least extreme option is the colonic massage, which involves a digestion-stimulating stomach rub. A more thorough approach is colonic irrigation, an invasive treatment in which the body's waste matter is literally pumped out of the system. For detoxification purposes this is second to none, but it's a serious procedure and shouldn't be undertaken lightly. Make sure the practitioner is licensed before going ahead with treatment.

feelgood factors

There's nothing better than indulging in a harmless bit of beauty frivolity in order to increase your glam factor and boost your mood. Here are some of the best quick and easy confidence-boosting tricks.

EIGHT WAYS TO FEEL GOOD

1. Shape up your eyebrows

This will 'open' your eyes and make your face look more expressive and possibly even younger (*see pages 76–77* to learn the technique). Start gingerly though – overly thin brows can look fake, especially if you've got dark hair. Also, you might notice a bit of redness after plucking, so try and do it the night before, not the morning of, a big day.

2. Try a new nail colour

It might be the oldest trick in the beauty book, but investing in a new nail colour can be one of the nicest treats you can give yourself. For a start there's the choosing – all those mini bottles lined up like colourful candies – and then there's the applying – a fresh coat of glossy colour on fingers or toes that will catch your eye whenever you glance towards them. Take your time to apply the colour, though – your 'mood lifter' might fast become a 'mood blackener' if you have to do it three times to get it looking right! *See pages 126–27* for a manicure guide.

3. Get shimmering

Sparkly body powders and lotions needn't be expensive – in fact, if you've got some shimmer powder for your face and some regular body lotion, you can make your own by mixing them together – but they'll definitely look it. Bare limbs become gleaming and gorgeous when treated to an added bit of sparkle – and don't worry about getting sticky, glittery bits everywhere. These days, formulations are so

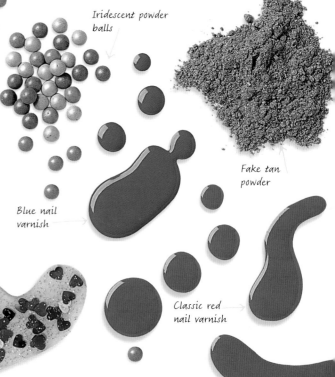

Iridescent powder balls

Fake tan powder

Blue nail varnish

Self-adhesive nail decorations

Classic red nail varnish

184

good that you don't have to go for a full-on 'tinsel' effect – many lotions just impart an iridescent sheen. They are especially good for use in the evening.

4. Soak yourself

Taking a bath isn't anything new, but this time, focus on the end result – not just getting a squeaky clean body, but a softer, smoother, more fragrant one, too. Add a few drops of softening bath oil to the water, plus a few drops of essential oils. Then while you're in the bath, buff and polish your skin with a loofah, body brush or exfoliator, paying close attention to elbows, knees and feet. The scrub will reveal fresh new skin and the oil will moisturise – so you'll emerge with baby-soft skin that will stay smooth all day.

5. Rev up your hair

Wash-in, wash-out hair colours are the saviour of those who are bored with their appearance. For a night out or a special occasion, they won't transform your hair colour but they'll 'lift' your existing shade so that it looks brighter and shinier and the natural highlights stand out more. Plus they come in individual sachets, so they don't break the bank, and most of them need to be left on for only five minutes, making them double quick to use, too.

6. Go fake

Adding a bit of colour to your face and legs can do wonders for your levels of confidence – it can make you look thinner, and it can also take the edge off that harsh, post-winter 'glare' that the skin can sometimes give off. If it's your first time out with fake tan, go cautiously with a thin layer of the product – remember that you can always build up the intensity over a period of several days. *See pages 152–53* for more useful information about fake tans.

7. New ways with old products

If your make-up bag is anything like most women's, it will contain at least one palette containing colours you have never used. If you're stuck in a beauty rut, it could be time you experimented with those cast-aside colours – particularly eyeshadow shades. Find out if you've got a 'warm' or 'cool' complexion by looking at your skin tone – if it's pink-based, you're cool; if it's yellow-based, you're warm. Cool complexions look better with blue-based shades, warm complexions are enhanced by peachy tones. But within that framework, your palette can be as wide as you like – you can get cool blues, greens and even pinks, for example – not to mention how great you'd look in metallic shades like silver. For warm tones, go for bronze, beige and brown shades as well as dusky greens, pinks and golds.

8. Copy a look

If in doubt, steal beauty tricks from someone else. Celebrities are a great place to start – they've often had the top make-up and hair people working on their look. Find a photograph in a magazine of a model or celebrity who you think looks great, then dig out some matching shades from your own kit bag.

Another good tip is to visit a beauty counter and single out the assistant whose look you most admire. You'll almost always find that her brand is the one that is most in keeping with your own style. Pick up some samples to try.

healthy body, happy life Is a better body the cause or effect of

a happy life? It can be both – so change your outlook and watch your body do the same. What are you waiting for? The sooner you begin, the sooner you will be able to welcome the new-look you.

HAVE FUN

If there's one thing that is guaranteed to help you remain steadfast on your path to a healthier body and a happier life, one piece of advice that will help you through – whether you're pushing yourself on the treadmill, preparing a super-healthy dinner or even discussing a body-changing operation with a cosmetic surgeon – it's this: relax and enjoy the experience.

There's no point in doing anything that's going to cause you stress, worry and unhappiness – that's a sure-fire way to ensure that you make the wrong decision or that your good intentions don't even carry you through to the end of the first week. No-one said that losing weight, getting fit or revitalising your body was going to be easy, but if you keep in mind that above all, it's supposed to be fun, you can rest assured that even the strictest routine will become a lot easier to stick to.

USE YOUR CREATIVITY

For a start, let's consider how to approach your diet. Don't make eating a miserable or guilt-ridden pastime. Let it be the social activity it's meant to be, by cooking dinner for friends, going out to restaurants and luxuriating over mealtimes – not bolting your food down as fast as possible. All restaurants have healthy options – dressing on the side,

two starters instead of a main course – so get creative with your ordering and you will be able to have the full and active social life you're used to as well as lose the weight.

Getting creative is something that applies to exercise, too: follow the old adage, 'if it feels good, do it'. Don't forget that hundreds of fun pastimes also constitute great exercise. Ice skating, roller blading in the park, dancing, cycling, taking a dog for an energetic walk, even playing 'catch the ball' with children – they're all great forms of exercise and ones that you're much more likely to stick to because you actually have fun while you're doing them.

Beauty rituals can also be great fun. There's nothing better than preparing for a night out with a group of girlfriends, swapping make-up tips and trying each other's creams and lotions. On your own, make chores like waxing and nail painting as pleasurable as possible by accompanying them with your favourite CD and preparing some delicious 'finger food' (so as not to smudge the polish!) like grapes, strawberries and nuts to have on the side.

THINK POSITIVE

As well as making your diet and workouts enjoyable, there are some positive things you can tell yourself that should cheer you up and spur you on. First, the longer you stick to your plan, the easier it gets. Soon you'll be racing around the block, bounding up the stairs and as for ice cream – who needs it? Second, it will all be worth it in the end. Just imagine yourself in that skimpy bikini, those new jeans or that stunning evening dress – and imagine the compliments and admiration from your friends.

Best of all, imagine how confident you'll be – ready to take on new challenges and put yourself in new situations. Start practising your new-found confidence today, and pretty soon you'll find that you're feeling better about yourself already, no matter where you are in your programme.

...AND RELAX

Finally, help yourself to feel good by ensuring that you're as relaxed and stress-free as possible at all times. The best way to feel relaxed is, of course, to feel rested – and that means getting your optimum number of hours' sleep per night. Don't forget that sleep is when cell renewal takes place. By the time we are thirty-five, our bodies begin to lose brain and other body cells at the rate of up to 7,000 per day.

Sleep gives our cell renewal systems a chance to regenerate, and it also lets us recharge our batteries for the new day ahead. Although each of us differs in the amount of sleep that we require, it's thought that if we all aim for around eight hours per night, our bodies should be able to keep themselves fighting fit. Also, if you go for a few nights with less than your minimum requirement, remember that it is possible to make up your sleep deficit around a week after – so giving yourself a lie-in at the weekend constitutes a health benefit as well as a relaxing treat.

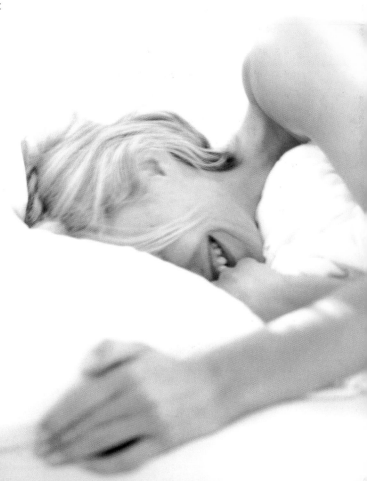

BED REST *Treat yourself to plenty of lie-ins: it's a great way of ensuring your long-term health and vitality.*

Contacts

British Allergy Foundation

Deepdene House

30 Bellgrove Road

Welling

Kent DA16 3PY

Tel: 020 8303 8583

www.allergyfoundation.com

British Association of Aesthetic Plastic Surgeons

34–43 Lincoln's Inn Fields

London WC2A 3PN

Tel: 020 7405 2234

www.baaps.org.uk

British Association of Plastic Surgeons

The Royal College of Surgeons

34–35 Lincoln's Inn Fields

London WC2A 3PN

Tel: 020 7831 5161

www.baps.co.uk

British Chiropractic Association

Blagrave House

17 Blagrave St

Reading

Berkshire RG1 1QB

Tel: 01189 505 950

www.chiropractic-uk.co.uk

British Dental Association

64 Wimpole Street

London W1M 8AL

www.bda-dentistry.org.uk

British Massage Therapy Council

Greenbank House

65a Adelphi Street

Preston PR1 7BH

Tel: 01772 881063

www.bmtc.co.uk

The British Medical Acupuncture Society

12 Marbury House

Higher Whitley, Warrington

Cheshire WA4 4AW

Tel: 01925 730727

www.medical-acupuncture.co.uk

British Nutrition Foundation

High Holborn House

52–54 High Holborn

London WC1V 6RQ

Tel: 020 7404 6504

www.nutrition.org.uk

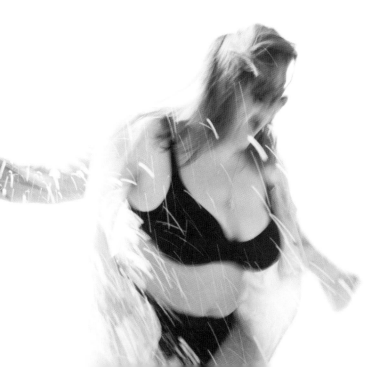

The British Reflexology Association

Monks Orchard

Whitbourne

Worcester WR6 5RB

Tel: 01886 821207

www.britreflex.co.uk

British Wheel of Yoga

1 Hamilton Place

Boston Road

Sleaford

Lincolnshire NG34 7ES

Tel: 01529 306851

www.bwy.org.uk

The General Osteopathic Council

176 Tower Bridge Road

London SE1 3LU

Tel: 020 7357 6655

www.osteopathy.org.uk

The International Federation of Aromatherapists (IFA)

182 Chiswick High Road

London W4 1TH

Tel: 020 8742 2605

www.int-fed-aromatherapy.co.uk

The National Back Pain Association

16 Elmtree Road

Teddington

Middlesex TW11 8ST

Tel: 020 8977 5474

www.backpain.org

National Osteoporosis Society (NOS)

Camerton

Bath BA2 0PJ

Tel: 01761 471771 (general enquiries)

Tel: 01761 472721 (for medical queries)

www.nos.org.uk

National Register of Personal Fitness Trainers

Thornton House

Thornton Road

London SW19 4NG

Tel: 020 8944 6688

www.nrpt.co.uk

The Pilates Foundation

80 Camden Road

London E17 7NF

Tel: 07071 781859

www.pilatesfoundation.com

The UK T'ai Chi Association

PO Box 159

Bromley

Kent BR1 3XX

Other useful websites

www.animated-teeth.com

Explanations and animations about these dental topics and procedures.

www.netdoctor.co.uk

Health information website

www.vitaminfo.com

Vitamin information service

www.spaaah.com

Spa directory

Index

Acknowledgements

The publisher would like to thank the following for the use of pictures:

IMAGE BANK / Nancy Brown 144 / Peter Cade 8 / Chris Cole 19, 113 / Ghislain & Marie David de Lossy 5, 80, 107, 118 / Britt Erlanson 60 / Rita Maas 140 / Nino Mascardi 12 / Hans Neleman 120 / Donata Pizzi 130 / Chris M.Rogers 25 / Simon Wilkinson 94

TAXI / Mark Adams 133 / Vincent Besnault 69 / Kaz Chiba 23 / Laura Lane 48 / Ken Reid 14 / Darren Robb 2 / Jeremy Samuelson 166 / Anne Marie Weber 47

STONE / Terry Doyle 143 / Erik Dreyer 103 / Holly Harris 169 /Chris Harvey 87 / Philip Lee Harvey 110 / JFB 155 / Ron Krisel 74 / Amy Neunsinger 159 / Kevin Mackintosh 66 / Stuart McClymont 43, 70–71 / Sean Murphy 98 /Peter Nicholson 28 /Jerry Racicot 153 / Thomas Schmidt 63 / Neil Snape 160 / Jerome Tisne 128 / Julie Toy 88 / Jane Wendell 57

Author acknowledgements

A whole army of devoted friends and family have been relentless in their provision of love, support and hot meals during the writing of this book. Thanks to Mum, Dad and Paul, Rachel, Colin, Elliot, Chris, Annabel and especially to Tommy, for being the nicest person in the world.

Thanks also to Sarah, Kate and Susanna, who have shared their knowledge and insights with me over the years, to Caroline for being such a fantastic editor and finally to Zanna Roberts, the greatest research assistant in the world, whose hard work, enthusiasm and attention to detail made writing the book an absolute pleasure.

Consultants: Nick Percival FRCS Consultant Plastic Surgeon; Dr Asker Jeukendrup, MSc Phd (nutrition); Harry Pearson, Health and Sports Therapist (fitness); John Groombridge, BDS (dentistry); S.A. Skaff (optometry); and Marilyn Sherlock, Institute of Trichologists (trichology).